Hope and Grace

of related interest

Spiritual Care in Practice
Case Studies in Healthcare Chaplaincy
Edited by George Fitchett and Steve Nolan
ISBN 978 1 84905 976 3
eISBN 978 0 85700 876 3

Palliative Care, Ageing and Spirituality
A Guide for Older People, Carers and Families
Elizabeth MacKinlay
ISBN 978 1 84905 290 0
eISBN 978 0 85700 598 4

Spiritual Care at the End of Life
The Chaplain as a "Hopeful Presence"
Steve Nolan
Foreword by Dr. Rowan Williams
ISBN 978 1 84905 199 6
eISBN 978 0 85700 513 7

Critical Care
Delivering Spiritual Care in Healthcare Contexts
Edited by Jonathan Pye, Peter Sedgwick and Andrew Todd
ISBN 978 1 84905 497 3
eISBN 978 0 85700 901 2

Talking About Spirituality in Health Care Practice
A Resource for the Multi-Professional Health Care Team
Gillian White
ISBN 978 1 84310 305 9
eISBN 978 1 84642 493 9

Making Sense of Spirituality in Nursing
and Health Care Practice
An Interactive Approach Second Edition
Wilfred McSherry
ISBN 978 1 84310 365 3
eISBN 978 1 84642 530 1

Hope and Grace

Spiritual Experiences in Severe Distress, Illness and Dying

Dr Monika Renz

Jessica Kingsley *Publishers*
London and Philadelphia

First published in 2016
by Jessica Kingsley Publishers
73 Collier Street
London N1 9BE, UK
and
400 Market Street, Suite 400
Philadelphia, PA 19106, USA

www.jkp.com

Library of Congress Cataloging in Publication Data
Names: Renz, Monika, 1961-
Title: Hope and grace : spiritual experiences in severe distress, illness and dying / Dr. Monika Renz.
Other titles: Hoffnung und Gnade. English
Description: Philadelphia : Jessica Kingsley Publishers, 2016. | Includes bibliographical references.
Identifiers: LCCN 2015039534 | ISBN 9781785920301 (alk. paper)
Subjects: LCSH: Terminally ill--Religious life. | Death--Religious aspects.
Classification: LCC BL625.9.S53 R4613 2016 | DDC 204/.42--dc23 LC record available at http://lccn.loc.gov/2015039534

British Library Cataloguing in Publication Data
A CIP catalogue record for this book is available from the British Library

ISBN 978 1 78592 030 1
eISBN 978 1 78450 277 5

Printed and bound in Great Britain

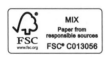

Experience at Night

I admit: I am hurt,
I stray,
exposed
to the mocking
and the walls of silence.

The freedom is mine,
arising on the narrow toeboard
of being loved,
to get to the heart of my suffering and to offer it
to the night itself, to the non-existent –

In the morning, I am 'found',
not knowing by whom,
by YOU.

Monika Renz

Contents

Acknowledgments

I am deeply grateful to everyone who has assisted me in my work, research, and publishing. My thanks go first to Prof. Dr. Thomas Cerny, Dr. Aurelius Omlin, Dr. Urs Hess, Prof. Dr Beat Thürlimann and Dr. Daniel Germann. I am indebted to my research assistant Dr. Miriam Schütt Mao, my study nurse Oliver Reichmuth, my colleagues Michael Péus, Anne Duveen and Dr. Christian Lenggenhager, my supervisor Dr. Gisela Leyting, the theologian Prof. Dr. Roman Siebenrock (Innsbruck), the hospital chaplains Klaus Dörig and Peter Gutknecht, the entire oncology team at St. Gallen Cantonal Hospital, and to my family. It is with the deepest respect that I express my sincere gratitude to the many patients at St. Gallen Cantonal Hospital, as well as the many participants in the further training programs I have offered on spiritual care, for sharing their intimate experiences with the sacred. It goes without saying that all the names in the book have been changed to protect the privacy of the individuals concerned. Special thanks go to my translator Dr. Mark Kyburz, to the editor of the German version of this book, Dr. Rudolf Walter, to Prof. Dr. Keith Anderson, and especially to Dr. Natalie Watson for her outstanding editorial support. My most personal heartfelt thanks go to my husband Jürg!

Introduction

"Where is God in human suffering?" Many patients ask this vexing question, so it became a major stumbling block, as well as an essential cornerstone of atheism, during the Enlightenment and ever since. Critical voices have asked, "How can God be good if he abandons us in suffering?" The concept of "God" has meanwhile been called into serious question. Fewer and fewer people think of God, let alone believe in him. Today, the most distinguished word for referring to God/the divine[1]—as a powerful influence and as a human experience of reality—is mercy or grace. Is there any grace in suffering? And how might this be related to hope?

The chasm between hope and grace is never greater than in suffering and illness. Nowhere does the meaning of life as

---

1   Patients have different approaches to God, to the divine, to the absolute, to a supreme being, to transcendence, or to a higher power. First and foremost, it is important to respect (patients') individual usage. Additionally, observing patients' spiritual experiences of transcendence suggests that it is important to distinguish two different aspects of the notion of God/the divine: the aspect of *relationship* and that of *being/the whole*. In this book, the term "God/the divine" first and foremost embraces all possible uses and individual notions, but emphasizes one concept or the other depending on patients' experiences. Various terms (experience of transcendence, experience of God, spiritual experience) describe one and the same phenomenon, but with different nuances (see Chapter 1).

a whole come under more intense scrutiny. And yet nowhere are hope and grace closer than in suffering and illness. Nowhere else does the unfathomable experience of God/the divine or of transcendence—also referred to in this book as spiritual experience—enter so frequently into the darkness of hopelessness and despair. Such deeply supportive experience is often long-awaited and yet utterly different than anticipated, after weeks or even months of bitter godforsakenness. Hope and grace are like courage and mercy, or what Ken Wilber calls "grace and grit" (Wilber and Wilber 1992/1996), a pair of words that bridge the gulf between the earthly and the divine.

Is grace, is salvation something we can achieve, something feasible, something we can buy? How? For centuries, a fierce debate raged in the Christian West as to whether salvation was to be achieved by good works, as asserted by the moralist Pelagius (c.390–418 CE), or whether it was entirely a matter of divine grace or mercy, a gift freely given, as maintained by his opponent Augustine of Hippo (354–430 CE). Martin Luther, the founder of the sixteenth-century Protestant Reformation in Germany, emphasized that salvation is by grace alone (*sola gratia*) thereby countering adverse developments in the Church at the time, which argued that salvation could be bought. This question has remained highly controversial to this day: can happiness, can serenity be self-made, or is it a blessing from a higher power, granted to us by the grace of God? The critically ill teach us that something truly fundamental occurs within them, exactly at the point where openness and grace converge. Finding an inner openness—be it only the determination to embrace the beauty of the day—involves emotional and spiritual hard work. Thus, we may ask, are happiness and serenity, perhaps, not an "accomplishment" after all? Can we nevertheless make them happen?

Grace is a gift from God/the divine, which is—in principle—always present. Neither God nor grace are here understood in dogmatic terms, but in terms of human spiritual experience. Grace can involve a profession of faith without, however, the rigidity of religious doctrine. Grace makes us more susceptible to something greater. And yet it either becomes experience or remains a construct.

To feel grace or not, to be connected or not, are the only alternatives. One and the same person may experience this connection as an inner reality, and a minute later feel disconnected again. Grace is another term for the divine, whether we call it God, a supreme being, the inconceivable, or the Whole.[2] Grace foregrounds the sense of a "gift" and concerns what we are unable to bring about ourselves. Grace and the "ego" are opposing qualities. Grace comes toward us and cannot be planned by the ego.

A dying mother who was very distressed about what would happen to her children after her death described her spiritual experience as follows: "I felt a lighthearted unconcern... solutions had been found, without me knowing what they were. But it wasn't simply 'nothing,' but everything."

Grace, as this example illustrates, always occurs differently than expected, in other categories and terms than anticipated.

A dying patient, who had gone hungry as a child during the war, had a vision of (his) paradise. He could not find the right words and thus began by saying, "I'll get more than a sandwich on the other side."

---

2   The notion of "God" needs to be distinguished conceptually from "the Whole," as that "which encompasses the whole while pervading its innermost sphere" (Hans Kessler, a spontaneous assertion made in private conversation). Whereas many people are barely able to overcome their aversion to speaking of "God," they have nevertheless experienced a state of being permeated by transcendence. The "whole" is a psychologically tangible word for God. By contrast, the word God resounds increasingly with an energetic dimension, a deliberate, goal-directed urging forward that is grounded in the whole (Renz 1996/2009: 281–4; Keller 2008). The present book cautiously attempts to approach what must ultimately remain an unnameable reality of being and its intrusion into our lives by way of various present-day experiences of transcendence.

Grace is thus experienced as a source of help from outside or from our innermost being.

This book starts out from *the* fundamental question of whether we can make happiness and serenity happen even amid suffering, or if they depend on mercy. It speaks of hope and grace. It explores what happens within the critically ill when, amid their suffering, they experience transcendence, a supreme being or "God as a reality within us." Traditionally, mysticism, in the different cultures and religions, talks about such experiences. But how do those who encounter transcendence now convey such experience? Time and again, even patients who have suffered for a long time report an indescribable sense of happiness, serenity, peace, or spirit when having such experiences. This book recounts such experiences (see Chapters 5 and 6), as well as what preceded them—for instance, a dream or a blessing. Besides reporting these experiences, this book also provides hard, tangible facts in the shape of categories and figures. Based on a research project involving 251 critically or terminally ill cancer patients ("Spiritual Experiences in Suffering and Illness": see Appendix), this book "counts" their many spiritual experiences of transcendence.[3] But why did the experience of the intangible, or of the numinous, happen to critically ill patients above all? The frequent nature of experiences of transcendence recorded during our project also surprised the participating physicians, nursing staff, and therapists. These findings offer hope to those who are suffering: spiritual experiences occur precisely amid suffering, namely,

3   The research gathered here was first published in Renz, *Grenzerfahrung Gott* (2003/2010); completely revised and published as *Hoffnung und Gnade* (2014b). The methodology and results were published in the *American Journal of Hospice and Palliative Medicine* under the title "Spiritual experiences of transcendence in patients with advanced cancer" (Renz *et al.* 2015). In this article and in the revised book (Renz 2014b), the earlier research and reports on patients have been completely restructured in terms of the current state of research. They have also been complemented with new patient examples.

when the ego's concepts and coping strategies have reached their limits. It is precisely here that grace seems to intensify and that a new openness begins to emerge (see Chapters 3 and 4).

No less promising and beneficial, according to our research, are the effects of spiritual experiences on patients' inner state, their attitude toward life and death, their fears and their pain. May one therefore conclude that happiness and serenity can be made and managed after all? Do religious persons, or those who practice meditation, live longer?[4] Are spiritual experiences— and thus their positive effects—reserved for religious persons? Do such experiences depend on religious affiliation or spiritual practice? Are spiritual experiences more common, for instance, among those who practice meditation? Our research suggests that such questions are neither expedient nor properly expressed (see Chapter 4). It is not a person's religious–spiritual *attitude* that seems to matter (King *et al.* 2013), but the *fact* that they do and how these experiences manifest. One key finding of our research is that such experiences of transcendence require openness and grace.

So what does the word "hope," one of the two words appearing in the title of this book, mean in this context? Hope, while implying openness, also suggests an inner orientation: ultimately, I argue, hope rests on grace and thus on the unexpected. The word circumscribes a state of mind and a fundamental stance characterized by a deep belief that one's life will eventually come to a good end.

For cancer patients, hope is a misleading word. Many cancer patients and their relatives "hope" for a miracle. Experience reveals that, on the contrary, they must leave behind—one step at a time—this unrealistic hope and discover a quality of hope, which amounts to something more, and yet something

---

4   The contemporary religion and health movement emerged from the USA and stressed a causal relationship between religion and health and funded research. This movement claims that religious persons cope better with stress, are happier, more optimistic, better integrated in society, and lead healthier lives (Koenig, King and Carson 2012).

else than a successful cure to their illness. Hope manifests itself in openness time and again. Yet this openness also has to be found. Hope is not a commodity that we *have* or possess. All we can do is to risk and to attain hope, time and again. Finding hope is a process, which can lead us through darkness, indeed through and beyond an often dreadful impasse, a nadir of suffering, to a new quality of existence, which in turn transcends the bounded ego (see Chapter 3). Hope is nurtured by the energy of vision, by grace. Etymologically, hope is related to *hopping*—that is, springing or leaping a short distance either once or in a succession of movements. We summon the courage to approach dimensions that would otherwise remain unexplored by hopping—by taking a leap of faith. Hope and grace complement each other, comparable to a couple. Hope arises from grace, and grace arises from hope. The mere fact that we are able to experience hope and a growing openness has already to do with grace (see Karl Rahner's theological approach to grace, Rahner 1984).

How, then, can we provide spiritual care and accompany patients in their spiritual processes between hope and grace? How can we support them in their waiting and struggling, their letting go and finding (see Chapters 3, 8 and 9)? How can we stand by the suffering when they are reduced to no more than perseverance for the sake of perseverance? Often they know God only in his absence, leading to a scornfulness that overshadows everything else. Many agnostic and atheist patients use the term "God" to stress his absence and deduce his inexistence from this absence. How do spiritual caregivers (such as pastoral caregivers, therapists, physicians, nurses, social workers, or volunteer carers) find the necessary circumspection? When should we insist on the religious question despite widespread reservations and the tendency of society to avoid such questions? Cicely Saunders (1918–2005), founder of the modern hospice movement, has recognized the problem of inadequate care in spiritual matters (Holder-Franz 2012). How, then, can we help others to interpret the intangible in a bold yet sensitive and non-manipulative way?[5] Over the years, patients have taught me that the sacred must be recognized for what it is, so as not to simply fade away and slip from consciousness. They have also taught me that caring about and preserving their spiritual experiences enhances their quality of life.

---

5   Here the question arises whether my own spirituality affects patients' experiences and interpretation. I am an open-minded religious person and a practicing Christian. I am attracted to a combination of religion, the depth psychology of C. G. Jung, Erich Neumann and Stanislav Grof, and to music therapy. Impressed by many encounters with patients, after some years of practice in psycho-oncology, I decided to broaden my background and studied theology at the universities of Zurich (Protestant), Innsbruck, and Fribourg (Catholic). I am also influenced by my studies in ethno-musicology, where I focused on healing rituals in different ethnic groups. I often have in-depth discussions and conversations with agnostics, who are not adverse to discussions of my approach to religion (Renz 2008a, 2013a, 2013b), to human development and to dying (see Appendix, Figures 10a and b). My deepest formative experiences occurred during bouts of illness when I was young and later after several accidents. What I experienced then was similar to a near-death experience and enhanced my sensitivity (e.g. for music, for vibration and for spirituality). My patients' deathbed visions, experiences of the transcendent and near-death experiences have influenced my special approach to theology, as several theologians agree. I differentiate three paths of interpretation of various holy scriptures such as the Bible: 1) there are words of revelation, written by humans inspired by a holy spirit; 2) there are passages that have to be interpreted from a historical-critical perspective, because they are influenced decisively by their historical context. These two approaches are common, but a third approach also has to be taken into account: 3) passages have to be interpreted on an (archetypal and/or culturally bound) *symbolic* level that corresponds to dream consciousness more than to rational everyday consciousness (see Appendix, Figure 10a). When these scriptures were written, people lived and thought naturally in terms of symbols and metaphors. Exactly this symbolic world seems to be analogous to the experiences and metaphors of the dying and of experiences in the liminal sphere of transcendence. Knowing about symbols and about the workings of the liminal sphere helps caregivers to better understand patients' specific use of language (see Chapter 2, see the list of metaphors of dying in Renz 2015). Otherwise patients wait and wait to be understood. Nonetheless, it is important in all spiritual care to raise the question of bias again and again (see limitations of our research in the methodology section).

Until now, *needs-based* spiritual care has attracted great attention among medical and healthcare professionals. One of the difficulties of this kind of spiritual care, which rests on an anthropological approach focused on human needs and resources, is that it is easily misunderstood as oriented toward wellbeing (programs).[6] Besides needs-based care and spontaneous compassion patients and their families need a therapeutic–spiritual approach based on a deeper understanding of the unconscious dimension, of dying as a transformation of perception comparable to a near-death experience (Lommel 2010; Renz 2015), and of spiritual, and, in turn, mystical experiences ("seeing as the mystics see," Rohr 2009). In other words, we need a profound knowledge of (archetypal) spiritual processes which occur when our everyday consciousness is transcended (see Appendix, Figure 10). My understanding of spiritual experiences, as well as of mental and emotional processes in the liminal sphere of our everyday consciousness and in the non-dualistic dimension ("non-dualistic thinking," Rohr 2009), enables a new quality of spiritual care. In dying processes, this means that a visible or invisible spiritual process and unexpected experiences of transcendence may occur within the dying even if patients called themselves non-religious before (see Renz 2015; see Appendix, Figures 5, 6 and 7). Thus, spiritual care is confronted with the difficult challenge of supporting the process and taking metaphors and signals seriously, but without any desire for religious manipulation. For all patients, dying and non-dying, process-oriented and experience-based spiritual care rests on the power of hope, of

6   In this book, "spiritual care" refers to the mental and emotional care provided by several professions in hospitals and nursing homes (see also Chapters 8 and 9). The term comes from the English-speaking world, where it is increasingly replacing pastoral care, as it is not connected with a specific religious tradition (Driedger 2009; Harding *et al.* 2008). In its introduction, the German online journal *Spiritual Care* speaks of "the shared responsibility of the health-care professions toward the spiritual resources and needs of the sick and their relatives" (www.spiritual-care-online.de; see also Roser and Borasio 2008; Frick 2009a; Weiher 2012).

keeping oneself open, and of expecting grace. It is precisely then that spiritual experiences often occur.

By no means does this kind of spiritual care contradict the therapeutic and pastoral focus on a patient's immediate needs and concerns (for instance, symptom control, pain management, and interpersonal problems). Crucially, however, we should not lose sight of the underlying, spiritual *process* that occurs in the liminal sphere of our everyday consciousness. So, we have to ask, what might a bodily symptom tell us about a *spiritual* process (see Cicely Saunders's often misunderstood notion of "total pain" in Holder-Franz 2012: 78–81)? What deeper longings do patients harbor, what energies drive and influence them, of what deeper desires do they still need to grow aware? Is there a difficult experience of primordial fear (see Renz 2015), or of inner darkness (see Chapters 2 and 5), which has been repressed and now wants to be addressed? And how can human beings deal with such fearful or dark experiences of the liminal sphere (Appendix, see Figures 10a and b). Is there, moreover, a slumbering experience of God himself, of the divine, or of transcendence that is waiting to enter consciousness? Precisely in dying processes, when patients are often no longer able to express themselves verbally, as well as in ineffable experiences of transcendence, the unconscious dimension is overwhelming. Thus, besides the needs-based knowledge an *indication-oriented approach* is called for, as practiced by our physicians Daniel Büche, Head of the Palliative Center, Florian Strasser, Head of Palliative Oncology, Thomas Cerny, Head of the Department of Oncology.

What qualifications do caregivers need to reach such an understanding of spiritual care? Which ones do end-of-life caregivers need in particular? Caregivers have to possess more than certain formal qualifications. Beyond specialized training, they must be willing to empathically endure the powerlessness of their patients, and to engage with their struggle through nothingness and their remoteness from God. Caregivers need to trust the spiritual–psychological process between fear and trust, struggle and peace, hope and grace. Moreover, they have to understand the principle of hope and final grace (see Chapters 3 and 4). Grace not only underpins but also reaches beyond therapeutic endeavor. Our task as caregivers is to create—and to keep open on behalf of our patients—the space in which "it may happen." In addition to the above aspects, end-of-life care needs to give particular attention to the patterns of the process of dying (transformation of perception, fears, struggles, difficulties in accepting, final maturation, the changing importance of relatives and family processes). Liminality and the laws by which it operates are predominant in the process of dying.

This book addresses pastoral caregivers, therapists, physicians, nursing staff and social workers, as well as the relatives of patients and laypersons interested in spiritual care. It offers guidance for approaching those who are suffering, for discovering their experience of the divine, of God and his absence (see Chapter 7). It provides some insights into the manifold expressions and effects of transcendence in our culture. It contains practical suggestions for providing spiritual and psychological care. In particular, this book proposes a new approach to spiritual care: in addition to needs and attitudes, it is based on spiritual processes (on a conscious and unconscious level) and on the occurrence of experiences of transcendence including experiences of darkness (see Chapters 8 and 9). Its undogmatic approach seeks to answer various fundamental questions about inter-religious dialogue and mysticism: should—or rather may—we ultimately conceptualize the divine as substance or as energy, as a Being or as a Thou? Should God or the absolute be conceived in terms of being or of relationship? In terms of the current debate on mysticism: Is our experience of the divine monistic or dialogic? This book adopts a both-and stance to these questions and illustrates its answers with a wealth of examples. Both being *and* relationship are important. They happen separately or together and simultaneously; both happen in the "One" (see Chapters 6 and 7).

Methodology and Background Research

The experiences with therapeutic–spiritual care reported in this book have grown from the palliative care I have provided to cancer patients and their relatives at the oncology divison of St. Gallen Cantonal Hospital, one of the largest oncology and palliative care centers in Switzerland. Among the inpatients and outpatients in my charge until late-2013 were over 1,000 individuals in the final stages of life and a comparable number of patients who recovered or went into remission. My work rests on a multidimensional approach to therapy. Patients are offered psychotherapy sessions, which include strategies for coping with illness, dream interpretation, family support, trauma healing, active imagination, music-assisted relaxation and spiritual care. I have developed this approach specifically for these particular patients, in order to do justice to their need for a stable relationship with the one and the same care provider, while undergoing changes with regard to their physical and mental health and oscillating states of consciousness. I am particularly interested in music therapy, which involves so-called music-assisted relaxation combined with active imagination. First, I give some verbal instructions for body awareness and relaxation, followed by entirely musical stimuli. My team and I work closely with palliative care physicians and nursing staff. Weekly cross-disciplinary consultations serve to determine which patients should be advised to have such therapeutic–spiritual assistance. Patients may, of course, accept or reject the support offered. Confidential issues remain strictly between patient and therapist.

Among those seeking spiritual care at our hospital are people of faith and those of no faith. Most of them have some kind of Christian background, though by no means all practice or attend church. Others are agnostics or atheists, and some are Muslims, Jews, Buddhists, Hindus, or adherents of folk religion. The religious attitude or spiritual practices of individual patients are sometimes recorded, and sometimes they are unknown at the beginning of spiritual–therapeutic care. Patients' emotional condition, the course of illness, pain, family distress, etc. are all of immediate concern. The spiritual dimension may come into focus or not; spiritual needs may be expressed or not; there may be no spiritual experiences at all, or they may intrude unexpectedly into "the here and now." Previous spiritual attitudes or experiences (for instance, through meditation, or near-death experiences) sometimes play a part, sometimes they do not. This particular therapeutic–spiritual care has been the subject of several research projects, which have been supported by the oncologists and palliative care specialists Dr. Florian Strasser, Dr. Daniel Büche, and Dr. Thomas Cerny, as well as by St. Gallen Cantonal Hospital (for instance, "Spiritual experiences of transcendence in patients with advanced cancer," see Renz *et al.* 2015).

Data collection

Over a period of one year, a prospective survey was carried out of all patients receiving palliative care over a shorter or longer period at our oncology division (N = 251). The survey was based on "participant observation," a method used in anthropology (Steinhauser and Baroso 2009) and ethnographic field research to study human behavioral patterns and tribal mindsets, as well as in the health sciences (Bluebond-Langner *et al.* 2007). Participant observation permits researchers to maintain professional distance while engaging empathically with patients, and to observe and record participants' use of language and context. Often, in this setting, the ineffable or self-evident in behavioral patterns and tribal mindsets enters awareness and finds verbal expression. We face the same challenge with the critically and the terminally ill, and with the suffering. In their emotional and spiritual processes, patients are at a loss for words. In their spontaneous experiences of transcendence, they speak of the ineffable *per se*. Participant observation grants patients the freedom to do as they wish, to share their experiences or not, to stammer, shout, cry, or—moved by the unfathomable—to remain silent. Patients are free to reveal their earlier life experiences or not, to hazard or suppress the path to increasing awareness. Participant observation further allows one to register small unambiguous non-verbal signals (for instance, nodding).

In our project ("Spiritual experiences of transcendence"), patients expressed their spiritual experiences; also, their associated reactions and preceding interventions or circumstances were recorded (see Appendix, Figures 3, 4 and 9). Notes were taken by the therapist after, but never during, therapy sessions. Most experiences were shared spontaneously. Sometimes, when the dimension of the transcendent resonanted implicitly (and hence unrecognized) through a patient's narrative, such as the sacred atmosphere of a dream, the therapist addressed this dimension cautiously, uttering her astonishment or sentiment (see Appendix, Figure 8). Does this not, however, amount to suggestiveness? This question is crucial, even more so in the case of critically and terminally ill patients. Ultimately, the question of manipulation calls for special attention (see also footnote 6). It demands caregivers be empathic with patients, to engage with their inner processes, and to be sensitive to the atmosphere. Every spiritual experience is personal and private. How can it be spoken about? As caregivers, we are allowed to offer patients a tentative interpretation of their (reported) experience, but they may of course reject this. However, patients often understand their own experience after such a tentative interpretation in a new way and react with astonishment. Quite a number of patients, in response to my suggestions, exclaimed, "That was grace!" In our project, these experiences were also recorded. Sixty-eight patients, including nine atheists, expressed a new attitude toward God/the divine, a new spiritual identity, and used the term "God" in this context at least once (see Appendix, Figure 3). They all experienced an "Aha!" moment, namely, that "he/it" had been involved.

Data analysis

Patient journals were analyzed and evaluated by two independent researchers using Interpretive Phenomenological Analysis (IPA). Where they disagreed, a third researcher was consulted. To interpret patient experiences and journals, as well as the signals they may have given unconsciously, as adequately as possible, we established a theoretical framework consisting of literature on near-death experience and mysticism on the one hand, and studies on symbolism and archetypes (especially Carl Gustav Jung and Stanislav Grof) on the other.

A follow-up study is currently underway at St. Gallen and Münsterlingen hospitals (both located in eastern Switzerland). Contrary to the research reported here, which is based on a single therapist's observations, the second study involves the observation of signals and processes of the dying—in particular their spiritual experiences or utterances in this direction—by the two palliative care teams (by nursing staff in the first instance and sometimes also by physicians, therapists, and hospital chaplains). Observations are made several times daily and recorded on corresponding sheets. These psycho-oncology and palliative care specialists are being assisted by international experts from the field of near-death experience (including Pim van Lommel), mysticism, theology and philosophy.

Chapter 1

Spirituality as Experience

The question whether God exists or not no longer stirs fierce debate. On the contrary, some argue that the question seems decided, at least in Western Europe. There is no verifiable evidence that God exists, nor can his existence be refuted. There is, however, one burning question regarding spirituality and *experience*: Can God, can the divine, can a higher power be *experienced*? Are such experiences credible/believable? Do they affect our lives, and if so how? And to whom can we turn with these questions in a culture and religion mostly deaf to such concerns? In what follows, I consider what people today—in particular the ill and the suffering—*experience* as God or as the divine, or indeed what they *lack* in the absence of such experiences of transcendence. Spirituality is a matter of human experience: the experience of the inconceivable.

Was that an Experience of Transcendence?

One initial experience triggered my understanding of spirituality. It began with the following dream: I was sitting in a small car. It was my car and yet it looked quite different. Suddenly a giant bear, standing ten meters tall, stood next to my car. He was about to devour me and the car, but failed. The event, and the horror, occurred three times during the dream. A hair's breadth from death, I was now safe at last. Beside me stood the wrecked car. Resolutely, I told myself: "I am going to drive myself, I am going to take matters into my own hands."

The next day, I flew off to a conference on spirituality. After my presentation, I was confronted with an unprecedented number of questions: Did I believe that God, that transcendence, could be experienced? Was what we experience as humans actually God, a supreme being, or just our imagination? After the conference, I was driven back to the airport through the evening rush hour on a three-lane highway. Suddenly, a vehicle traveling at maximum speed came headlong toward us, barely missing us. Our car skidded—from left to right, and then to the left again... Then there was nothing but light, blinding light. Finally, our car came to a standstill, almost at a right angle to the traffic. A bus came thundering toward us and managed to brake just in time. Our car was still roadworthy. I climbed out of the backseat and said: "Right, I am going to drive now." When I bid farewell to my companion at the airport, I glanced back at the car and was startled: the car in my dream had looked similar.

Was this an experience of transcendence, of God? What should I make of it? How could I understand my dream? I was shaken for days. One thing that I have been aware of ever since is: spirituality has to do with something "huge" (the giant bear in my dream), something of a magnitude that eludes the categories of human understanding. Dealing with this greatness requires autonomy (the symbol of the car in the dream) and an ego capable of governing. The experience made me thoughtful. I would be either foolhardy or a staunch atheist not to believe it. Conversely, I would be a religious fanatic not to allow myself to doubt and to adopt a dispassionate distance.

Norbert, a dying patient in his mid-fifties, did not know whether to consider himself a Christian or a Buddhist. Although he had said his farewells, he could not die. For two weeks, he simply lay on his bed for the sake of being, as he told me once. Music played on the monochord touched him even though he did not know what was happening to him. There was nothing but sound, which had shaken him like the waves of the sea. He had never heard such sensuously simple music. Yes, it was the music, but also a great deal more: "The music ensured there was something. As if I could hear the atmosphere vibrate." "Did you sense a presence?" I asked him cautiously. He pondered this question for days and slipped more and more into a different state of consciousness, at times barely within reach. The sound of the monochord touched him a second time, prompting the following comment: "That sound with the overtones is like a heavenly tent, into which I either fall or fly. Whether falling or flying makes no difference. It is all the same. Just like being a Christian or a Buddhist. All that matters is presence! Something is here, and I am here, but soon no longer." Norbert became increasingly reticent. The atmosphere surrounding him deepened in his final hours. He died peacefully, and in the end took the secret of his identity with him.

Karin, a childless academic alienated from the Church, grew worse every day. One of our first conversations was about relationship problems and her difficulties with being touched. Now she lay on her bed with her eyes wide open, in obvious pain, suffering from shortness of breath and a panic-stricken fear of the intensive care unit. I encouraged her to be guided into music-assisted relaxation, actively imagining that she were guiding a ray of light through her body. I encouraged her to observe where in her body the light was received, where it was less and to establish where this experience was pleasant and where less so. While uttering no religious words, she described what had evidently been a dense experience: "The angels were close. The light grew larger; it came from outside and resembled Jesus, who said to me: You will survive, just let it happen." After a further operation, she asserted: "The light was also in the intensive care unit; it was like a near-death experience."

My discussions with Alain were intense. There was never any mention of God and faith, until one day he heard that I was also a trained theologian. He had no interest in God and organized religion, which for him were fraught with morals, too many wars and too much suffering. God meant nothing to him, but he was a passionate organist. At some point, he asked me what God meant to me. Following my spontaneous reply, I asked him what he experienced when he played the organ. "Oh, there is no way of telling." I told him about God at Mount Sinai, how Moses had experienced God as so powerful and numinous that neither words nor images had existed to describe him. Perhaps playing the organ was just as indescribable. Alain interrupted me: "Are you saying that what I feel when playing the organ is an experience of God?" "I imagine so." Silence. Moved, he said: "It is truly inexpressible." Touched by his words, I insisted: "Strong emotion is part of the great experience because within us occurs something that exceeds us." In the following weeks, our conversations intensified. Alain wanted to hear more, and even to pray. During those final weeks, he grew more confident, defying all his fears.

One Phenomenon, Different Names

While describing something similar, the phrases "the experience of transcendence," "spiritual experience" and "the experience of God" have particular nuances:

The experience of transcendence, deriving from Latin *transcendentia* (literally, a climbing over), denotes what is induced by such experiences and what lies beyond them. Thus, in the previous examples, patients report how they are existentially moved, how their body and soul are intrinsically touched, and how they experience a religious moment, which in effect opens them up to another—divine or sacred—dimension. Whereas palliative care commonly refers to the experience of transcendence as referring to the spiritual experiences of atheists in particular (McGrath 2005), this book has another, wider focus.

The experience of God: Many people recoil from this term, some because they are caught within their aversion to God, others out of (religious) respect, because they would prefer this ultimate word to remain a mystery than hear it uttered (Rahner 1969). This book highlights a third reason why "the experience of God" is eschewed: behind the rejection often lies the primordial human experience of the numinous, which we must imagine as absolute, skin-piercing, and thus as deeply imperative and overwhelming. Our diminuitive ego encounters God almost "bodily," as a tremendous infinite Whole (I have discussed the primordial fear in Renz 1996/2009: 49–61; see also Renz 2015). As mentioned above, I experienced a gigantic bear and a blinding light. Other people dream of elephants (a sacred animal in India, by the way). The term "experience of God" stresses the aspect of encounter in contrast to aspects of being (*unio mystica*) or energy. It focuses on a relationship with him (God or a supreme being) and thus reminds the ego of the unbridgeable difference between a small defenceless human being and an incomprehensibly large "Other." At times, this Other is experienced as protective, redemptive or life-giving, at others as menacing to the point of being overpowering. From this threat has sprung—and still springs—a fundamental taboo: God himself, or the holy, is taboo, both in his experential aspect and as a numinous Other. For centuries, the experience of God, or rather the idea that God himself could be experienced, was banished from ecclesiastical teaching. Only mystics, from their independent position on the margins of society, believed that God/the divine could be experienced. No less suppressed today is the aspect of a binding commitment. Whenever the *experience* of God is at issue, we are much more strongly connected and challenged to adopt a binding, responsive stance, in contrast to "merely" speaking of the divine, the cosmos, a higher power, a supreme being and the experience of being. Only few people are simply open: either to an experience according to their own religious tradition (Judeo-Christian, Muslim, Buddhist, etc.) or to a totally different experience. The term *experience of God* stresses the absolute, the powerful, but also the unsettling aspect of such experience. The present-day non-committal understanding of spirituality stems, so it seems, from an aversion to the term God, and therein from our deep uncounsious primordial fear.

Spiritual experience: The word "spiritual" has various meanings today, stretching along the broad spectrum between holistic "wellbeing," the expansion of consciousness, and mysticism. In the history of concepts, spirituality—more than religiousness— denotes *experience* and stands for the experiential dimension of religion. *Spiritualis* is the Latin cognate for the Greek *pneumaticos* and means "woven by the Spirit" (*geistgewirkt*). The verb *pneo* means to breathe, to blow, to smell. In the second century CE, *spiritualis* meant the inner experience had—or indeed not had— by the baptized adult during the rite of baptism. In terms of the history of concepts, this experience evolved more and more into a particular religious attitude and piety. The testimonies of monks, desert fathers and mystics bear witness to the fact that spirituality stood for a life born from the Holy Spirit. The word *spiritualité* appeared again in the French language after 1700. Then it meant a personal relationship with God. Even if by now we talk about spirituality as an attitude, the original experiential aspect should not be forgotten. Spirituality is indeed a synonym of the experience of God/the divine. The nineteenth-century psychologist of religion William James (1811–1882) spoke of a personal religious experience whose roots and center lay in mystical states of consciousness (1902/1979: 358).

This book applies the various terms (experience of transcendence, experience of God, spiritual experience) to one and the same phenomenon, depending on the nuance. The aforementioned study (Renz 2015) refers to spiritual experience throughout. However, more important than names and labels are the characteristics of the phenomenon and a growing sensitivity to caring. Spiritual care, then, focuses not primarily on different religions and their beliefs, but on the phenomenon of subjective experiences of transcendence, which can deepen or enlarge one's own attitude.

The Characteristics of Experiences of Transcendence

Key to our study are the following characteristics of spiritual experience (see also Renz 2007: 40):

- *Spirituality is experiential* (Sudbrack 1999). There can be no spirituality without experience. Spirituality is a liminal occurrence. *Spiritual experience happens at the limits of the ego* and at the limits of the world known to that ego, in its transition from one mode of perception to another (Renz 1996/2009; see also Renz 2015). Arnold and Lloyd (2013) identify the transformation of perception as one of the four categories of experiences of transcendence. I distinguish between experiences of God/the divine as the absolute and ultimate in contrast to experiences of the liminal sphere (see Chapter 2). This sphere is shaped by altered perception. Here, patients have wonderful, angelic experiences, as well as experiences of darkness and transition (see Chapter 5).

- *Spiritual experiences or experiences of transcendence bear witness to an utterly different quality of being, of a category that is not bound by space, time or causality, nor by corporeality.* Near-death experiences, for instance, are explained in terms of the presence of nonlocal and endless consciousness (Lommel 2010; Fenwick 2010). This other category of existence accounts for the intensity of spiritual experience. There is a heightened sense that we have a home elsewhere, in another world or state of being. Spiritual experiences induce desire.

- *Spirituality intimates a relationship between the human being and the sacred/God/the divine.* Spiritual experiences set us free and connect us at the same time. We are free from the ego-centered mind, thoughts, and emotions, from fears and obsessions, free to be ourselves. The dying often feel freer than ever before, free *from* themselves and free *toward* themselves. But spiritual experiences also bind us, essentialize us, connect us, and make us, in particular, auditively sensitive (see Chapter 4). To speak of a relationship is somewhat bold, however, because we always know only one side, namely, ours. Spirituality affords us a glimpse of an ultimate connectedness with God/the divine (see Chapters 5 and 6).

- *Spirituality is a moment of transcendence amidst the everyday as well as amidst the magnificent* (see Chapter 4). Spiritual experiences occur amidst the unremarkable and the extraordinary, within the context of groundbreaking insights and pioneering creativity, amidst sensory impressions, dreams, common everyday events, love, and our search for meaning. Extending beyond the everyday, these experiences offer us something special. Spirituality is what transcends and reveals and what makes the everyday deeply meaningful.

- *Spirituality is a gift of grace.* Theology speaks of revelation. Spiritual experiences bear witness to mystery. To some extent, they remain mysterious and elusive. We can never make or trigger them, we cannot prescribe or take them as a drug. Instead, they occur unpredictably, only to vanish no sooner have they appeared. I often compare them to a loose electrical connection.

- *Spirituality is an energetic occurrence.* We are most likely to experience the energetic aspect of God/the divine through the effects of spiritual experiences. Such experiences have an inherent urgency—they prise open the familiar, connect the tension-filled, establish peace, and effect reconciliation. Their energetic feature, such as the synchronicity of inner and outer events, is not harmless.

- *What is needed is a strong personality and an ability to experience awe.* The utterly different and numinous nature of spiritual experience, as well as its concomitant effects such as the disappearance of pain, astonish us or make us shudder. From the fact that the angel in the Bible often says "Fear not (Do not be afraid)" (Luke 1.13, 30; 2.10) we can deduce that there must be a sphere that evokes anxiety. Given their characteristics, spiritual experiences elude full understanding, leaving us with just limited scope for integration. Keeping in touch with reality is crucial during such experiences. This highlights a difference with psychosis. Only the strong, governing personality is able to perceive spiritual experiences without fragmenting and accept them as true. After every experience, we need to ground ourselves (see, for instance, the descent from the holy mountain in Matthew 17.1–9). This helps us to find our way into an inner distance. On the other hand, we need to recall the experience itself from time to time, for instance, through rituals—the term echoes the original meaning of "liturgy." (On dealing with spiritual experience, see Chapters 8 and 9; on integration, see Scagnetti-Feurer 2009.)

Beyond Fear and Bodily Symptoms

Time and again, spiritual experiences lead into a sphere beyond fear. In our project, 75 out of a total of 135 patients who had one or more spiritual experiences reported a freedom from anxiety. A similar number (71) experienced pain relief to the point of freedom from pain. How are we to explain this deliverance from fear? We experience pain and personal needs only if they are the rudiments of an ego and if we are concerned about something that we call our own. Plants express "personal" needs by reaching up toward light and by requiring water. But beyond this ego-centered mode of being, there is no fear. Beyond fear, we no longer seem to be caught up in our pains and symptoms. Precisely this is what patients teach us during and after their experiences of transcendence. They describe peace, being, bliss, reverence. Meditative immersion or holotropic breathing can open up our awareness to the point of a perception beyond body and ego. Meditating Buddhist monks exhibit stronger high-frequency gamma waves on a magnetic resonance tomograph, indicative of an enhanced level of attention and concentration. Also evident among these monks is greater activity in the left frontal cortex, a sign of "cheerful equilibrium and peace of mind" (Lutz *et al.* 2004; Kraft 2005).

> *Andrea, a dying woman about 50 years old, was desperate. She asked me how she could take her own life. "This is not a life, it is an insult!" Sharing her despair, I returned her gaze. "You are desperate because you can no longer do what you want and used to enjoy. However, I prefer the word imposition to insult. Your life has become a brutal and harsh imposition. Is that true?" My remark caught her interest. She understood that the term "imposition" also dovetailed with her strength of character and her perseverance. She smiled briefly before engaging in further reflection. Then, a jolt went through her body, her ego once again took hold of her, and she repeated: "I still want to kill myself though; I do not want to be in this condition." I breathed heavily and said: "There is almost nothing I can say. I myself would probably be just as desperate in your situation. But I believe there is an alternative to your miserable condition. Not that there is much that I can tell you about that alternative. However, you can experience this from within, maybe with the help of deep music-assisted relaxation, what I call a 'Journey in Sound'. Would you like to try this?" Andrea expressed interest and so I introduced*

relaxation exercises to intensify her body awareness for one part of the body after another, accompanied by the soft sounds of a lyre, until eventually there was nothing but sound. Already during the music, I sensed intensity, timidity, even spirituality in the room. Andrea lay there for hours, her arms spread, her breathing calm. That evening, she thanked me: "I felt weightless, as if I were far away, and yet in the here and now. The limits of my body had gone. There was no pain, no anger, no fear. What could it have been?" She had tears in her eyes. I asked her whether things had somehow felt sacred. "Yes, absolutely, but why?" Did "God" mean anything to her? Had God been present? She nearly yelped: "Oh yes, that was the special aspect. It was HIM, so extensive, so great." Andrea was deeply moved and free of pain for days. Suicide was no longer an issue. "Amidst this greatness killing myself is out of the question. I don't know why, but it's not right, it's just not done," she told me.

Later, when she was about to be transferred to a nursing home, she was once more overcome by despair, pain and suicidal thoughts. She considered herself too young to be admitted to a nursing home, where patients did nothing but slurp their soup. We looked at each other silently. "You wouldn't want to go to the nursing home either! But perhaps I ought to ask that other state, and see what it tells me." Once again, Andrea had a spiritual experience during music-assisted relaxation. Deeply moved, she said: "Again, I simply don't understand. But there is a solution." Later, she told me that she would never understand God: "But I have experienced, I have heard his word: 'Be of good cheer.'"

This patient's contact with the great God/the divine illustrates what I mean, when I compare the relationship to God/the divine to a loose electrical connection: sometimes patients feel connected, at other times they don't. While the other side of the relationship—God, a supreme being, the Whole, the light, in my eletrical metaphor the power network—is permanently related to us, "on standby," and offers us the opportunity to establish contact, we are able to connect only intermittently. Only in times of openness and grace can we hear the atmosphere of the sacred. But what happens when that loose connection with God/the divine breaks off? And how do experiences in the liminal sphere border on experiences of transcendence, immediately before and after the connection just described?

Chapter 2

Between Two Worlds

The Liminal Sphere and Its Laws

This book refers to the region *bordering on* transcendence as the "liminal sphere." Here, in this "border region," we are not yet or no longer aware of actual participation in the divine. But neither are we any more within our normal, ego-based, subject-related perception (as we feel and perceive immediately as an ego with sensations, instincts, needs and ideas). Instead, we find ourselves in limbo, in a situation perhaps best described as a "neither/nor" or as a "not only/but also."

Three Examples

Hannah was exuberant and peaceful. She asked me, "Where am I now?" Only moments earlier, she had trembled with fear.

Peter, a man from a humble background, was deeply moved by his music-assisted relaxation, which had been accompanied by the sounds of a harp: "The atmosphere was indescribable— sheer bliss." The next day, he requested another music-assisted relaxation. *This time I played the monochord for him. Overwhelmed by his sadness about his condition and by his loneliness and by feeling cold, he asked me to abstain from playing music. He would be unable to bear the feelings that might then burst forth.*

Months later, after his readmission to hospital, we had several good encounters. He wanted to talk about God and the world. One morning, he revealed his deep distress: he had dreamed several times about being ensnared, sucked into a vortex, by an evil woman. This vortex, which resembled a funnel, was butchering him to pieces. Only at the very end was he unexpectedly rescued. Then he felt "whole again" or indeed "safe." He told me that he had had the same nightmare as a young child. Peter's account suggested a sense of "being at the border," catapulted back into an earlier traumatic state that had caught up with him again in his illness. I asked him whether he could tell me about his childhood, whether there had been a place or a person where he had felt particularly at ease. "Oh, yes, on my father's knee, the world was fine! But I never liked—and I still really don't know why—being in my aunt's kitchen upstairs. I was always on my guard there." We both felt devastated and fell silent. Then I asked him: "Could you, the adult Peter, imagine traveling back in your mind to young Peter in order to protect him?" "Yes, I could," he said, "but I don't know exactly how." I asked him to close his eyes and to imagine us both going toward young Peter. I ask him "Is that okay?" "Yes. We've reached him, but he's afraid," he told me. "For me," I say, "there is something like God that is greater and stronger than any fear. In earlier times, people used to be blessed to receive God's protection. Would Peter like to be blessed too?" Peter nodded. Almost aghast at my own courage, I heard myself saying that God's protection could liberate us from this fear. Before me, I saw a small boy, sweating. Then I spoke the following words into the tense atmosphere: "Hello Peter. The adult Peter and I, Mrs Renz, are here to see you. We have come to rescue you from this kitchen and to bless you.

Peter, you are protected and safe. Whatever evil happens, will pass you by. Deep within yourself, you are wholly protected. Can you hear me?" "Please could you repeat these words. Peter is listening carefully, but he doesn't understand," Peter, talking about himself in the third person, asked me with his eyes still closed. I asked if he would like me to make the sign of the cross on Peter's forehead, as a sign of protection? "Oh yes." The gravity of the situation dawned on me and my throat thickened. Was this the distress that this man had suffered as a child? I made a gesture to indicate that I was going to touch him, then made the sign of the cross on Peter's forehead, and said: "Peter, you are protected, also in this awful kitchen. No matter how afraid you are, you have God's blessing." Now I asked Peter whether he wished to find words or say a prayer, to prove to himself the seriousness of the moment. "Yes... Our Father..." His prayer was followed by the sounds of a harp, then silence, before Peter said softly: "Ah, that's good. Peter is sitting on father's knee. The kitchen isn't that bad any more." Ten nights without nightmares ensued.

Elias, a man of distinction, told me about a near-death experience that he remembered during his stay in hospital. "I'm not religious, but..." He had almost died after that operation. He had seen a kind of ethereal light, white and yet bluish, absolutely magnificent. It soothed him to think of this light. His pain then faded away. During a breathing exercise, I encouraged Elias to behold and breathe in this light. Suddenly he shot up: a step beneath the magnificent altar, things had not been beautiful at all. His old enemies, from his primary school days and from his life in business, had come and mocked him. He had felt ashamed. And there was a terrible noise. "Then, suddenly, this all seemed gone. An angel stood on the right, and I climbed up and saw the altar, surrounded by incense. By and by I saw nothing but this wonderful white and bluish light. I shuddered, it was so beautiful! I have asked myself ever since, with quite some astonishment, 'who' is this light?"—It occurred to me that Elias did not ask, "What was this light?" but "who?" (See the experience of the Other in Chapter 6.)

The Characteristics of the Liminal Sphere

What is the nature of perception in the liminal sphere? Liminal experience follows certain general patterns even though perception is still individually shaped:

a) *A dominant sense of creatureliness*: an acute awareness of oneself as only a small creature in relation to creation, the creator, all-or-nothingness. One example is Job 10.9: "Remember that you fashioned me like clay and will you turn me to dust again?" Another is the ashing ritual on Ash Wednesday: "Remember that you are dust, and to dust you shall return." (see Genesis 3.19)

b) *A closeness to the divine*: the numinous Thou has become irrepressible.

c) *The ambivalent nature of experience*: experiences of beauty and of paradise stand side by side with a near-total sense of threat, forlornness, darkness.

d) *A sensitivity to angels and an angelic atmosphere* (recorded among 66 patients in our study; see Chapter 5), as well as to *demonic figures and dark energies*: good stands side by side with evil (e.g. experiences of the vortex, the darkness of near-death experiences). In our project, 56 patients had profoundly beautiful spiritual experiences along with experiences of struggle and darkness (see Chapter 5; Appendix, Table 1).

e) *Energy sensitivity*: Good and bad energies are "felt," indeed sometimes so consciously that some people believe that they are experiencing brain wave activity: "My head feels different," "My head feels really tight, and then wide-open," "I feel hunted, then free."

f) *Vibrational and auditive sensitivity:* Patients are noticeably receptive to music, to atmospheres, and to an authentic tone of voice (or its absence). Music is the medium closest to a threshold in consiousness; music is prevalent in human liminal sphere perception.

g) *A closeness to formative influences and childhood experiences:* Children move back and forth between waking, dreaming, and sleeping, often entering and then remaining in the liminal sphere. Correspondingly, in adults this sphere reactivates childhood feelings of confidence and trust, safety and security, but also the fears and the speechless distress we suffered as small children. In the liminal sphere, the world of symbols of which we had an instantaneous grasp as children once again moves closer and becomes "real." (Peter: "Sitting on my father's knee, the world was fine.")

h) *Psychological nakedness:* Mechanisms of ego defense, self-assertion, and control functions become irrelevant; without repression and its protective armor, the ego is as it were psychologically naked (and experiences feelings of shame). This nakedness becomes an imposition (we are exposed to our inner states and fears), but it also presents the opportunity for the greatest possible transformation (near-death experiences, for instance, allow us to start life from scratch again). To be naked means to feel ashamed, but also to be close to one's personal essence.

On the whole, liminal experience is completely alien to our usual subjective and subject-related, ego-centered existence. In the liminal sphere, we are more dependent than ordinarily. We are easily irritable and stressed, but also grateful, receptive to touch, and often overcome by happiness and sadness. I have observed this among the critically ill, patients in rehabilitation, persons awakening from a dream or anesthesia, and those who have had a near-death or deep meditation experience. Children, artists and the elderly repeatedly experience this perception of the liminal sphere and its workings. They oscillate between the "here and now" and an utterly different sphere, which I elsewhere describe as ego-distant (Renz 2015), and they experience in-betweenness.

Liminal experience eludes the grasp of everyday perception. Nevertheless, it should neither be degraded as sentimentalism nor as an estrangement from our basic essence. On the contrary, such experience is profoundly authentic (as the saying goes, "children and fools speak the truth"). Amidst such experience, we can barely escape from ourselves. Even profound emotions such as sadness, fear, or shame are beautiful because they cannot lie.

Here, the ego is also close to the numinous and aware of its own weakness. Here begins not only our astonishment but also our shrinking in the face of the greatness of creation, the creator and the ultimate order of things. Now approaching an entirely different mode of perception (because it lies beyond our established categories of space, time, causality, corporeality and bodily symptoms), not only do we see differently, but we also see different things. Liminal perception moves us closer to an utterly different—and inexplicable—reality of being.

In the liminal sphere, however, we find ourselves *not yet quite* or *no longer quite* "within" that other state of being. At the limits, both worlds are present, at times irreconcilable, at other times overlapping. This explains the emergence of mixed phenomena and mixed perceptions in this transitional stage: the dying, as an expression of their altering sense of gravity, are afraid of falling into a bottomless abyss. Our dreams, but also folktales, are peopled with frightening or caring figures. Whereas our anxiety indicates our ego-bound feelings, in this transitional region we lose our subjective, self-centered or ego-bound ability to differentiate our surroundings. What emerges in their place is a similarly blurred scenario that may culminate in the numinous. The liminal sphere is where subjective perception either begins or once again dissolves, where supernatural opposites, forms and images become real. Dreams are common in the liminal sphere. Thus it is hardly accidental that dream consciousness is widely understood as a state between the unconscious and consciousness. The greatest possible transformation takes place precisely in this liminal sphere. From here a new beginning may unfold, as confirmed indirectly even by recent neurobiological findings on religious experience. Hüther (2004), for instance, found that coping with stress reactions to internalized beliefs (that is, "still being able to believe") has a similar effect to interpersonal closeness (reduced release of stress hormones, activation of positive endogeneous transmitters). If, however, uncontrolled stress reactions occur, such as in liminal experiences and panic attacks (when our previous problem-solving strategies are defunct), old neural connections may be broken and in their place new, more complex synaptic connections may establish themselves. In religious terms, a crisis, in which our conceptions of God/ the divine collapse, may lead to our exploring new possibilities and opening up new paths: "God comes into play when we must cope with fear, when our previous notions are broken" (Jaschke 2013: 61).

On the one hand, the beginnings of life, that is, the early development of consciousness and, on the other hand, those stages of life in which ego-consciousness once again becomes fragile, are characterized by liminal experience. In nearing death, and in out-of-the-ordinary situations, people often have liminal experiences that bring back the memory traces of times long gone and spheres far away. Here, the inner child, the internalized, supernatural figure of the mother (for instance Mary, the mother of Jesus/God, or maternal goddesses), the power animal and angels appear as spiritual guides. Angels, to be understood as messengers, open up our path to the essence and to the divine (for instance, the appearance of the altar, incense, and the ethereal light in Elias's dream). Although not identical, God/the divine is indirectly present when an angel appears to us. Angels are the celestial "messengers" between God/the divine (see Chapter 5) and human beings.

Surrounded by Music and Vibrations

Whereas adult life is determined chiefly by the visual and rational perception of the world, in the liminal sphere another mode of perception becomes central. Liminal states are "hearing"—auditive—states, in which we are *connected* to the world as a surrounding whole. Our visual and rational *engagement* with the facts of the world contrasts with our hearkening for the mystery. However phrased, in the womb, in dying, in a coma, in deep regressions, and in experiences of transcendence we are receptive to presence and vibrations and auditively connected to a totality of sound. Physically, our presence and our surroundings are vibration, sound, and atmosphere.

I speak of the auditive phases of life, in which we hear *differently* and hear *other* things. Luban-Plozza (2000: 839) observes that there is:

> verifiable evidence for the auditory perception of our surroundings beginning already during the intrauterine phase… Everything suggests that the actual code of sound-related expression establishes itself during this lifephase… The ability to recognize the emotional content of different tone of voice and language undoubtedly develops already during this stage of human existence.

I speak of a transformative experience of music (Renz 1996/2009, 2015).

During such auditive phases of life, we experience ourselves as "inside" (within the vibrational totality) rather than as separate or "off-key." We "do not stand above things," but are a part of a larger whole. We are determined by being, rather than by doing, and by ourselves. Being-inside means being powerless—without any power of our ego—and as such dependent. For the growing fetus and also for the critically ill, a certain mood or atmosphere, a tone of voice perceived to be more or less authentic invoke an experience of the world and of the self. Correspondingly, we are (totally) irritated by an uncomfortable atmosphere, caused, for instance, by conflicting messages and double binds (*Doppelbotschaften*). Children initially feel a need to get more and more love, nurture and comfort, out of a need to compensate. But if compensation fails, more and more psychological damage may occur (Lempp and Becker 1984; Herzka and Jeanrenaud 1986). Critically ill patients exhibit signs of emotional conflict and emotional forlornness. Many cease to respond to their surroundings, as they are getting closer to death. Is this a protective reaction?

Our dependence on hearing is an opportunity for music therapy. Music gains particular importance in caring for patients in liminal states and thus in auditive phases of life (Renz 1996/2009: 31–6). Music reaches us where we are otherwise beyond reach. It subverts our fears and our closely guarded narcissism, softens hard edges, and soothes distress. Music experience reaches us deeper than words. Music, then, is a primary kind of resonance chamber. In the terminology of C. G. Jung, music reaches deep archetypal material (Luban-Plozza 2000: 839; see Appendix, Figure 10a).

Silence is also part of music. Music is limited neither to classical music such as that of Mozart, nor to folk music, pop or jazz. Music therapy, especially with critically ill patients, focuses on individual tones, melodies, archaic rhythms, monochromatic sounds, and their effects. Music-assisted active imagination and relaxation usually begins with guided body awareness and relaxation. Visual stimuli sometimes evoke active imagination and gradually give way to exclusively musical impulses.

No other medium is closer to spirituality than music. Music is both real and intangible, as is spirituality. Music is the medium furthest removed from our everyday consciousness and nearest to a threshold in consiousness. This explains why music is the prevalent medium of the liminal sphere and reaches our most profound fears and desires. Music subverts our ego defense and boundaries, music opens us to the transcendent (dimension of sound) and grounds us again (dimension of rhythm). All this explains its widespread use in shamanic rituals across the world to induce an altered state of consciousness and to subsequently guide the entranced person back to the earthly "here and now." In the aforementioned study, 98 patients had a spiritual experience during or after music-assisted active imagination.

The Liminal Sphere and the Beginning Division Between Good and Evil

God/the divine always have to be conceived as substance, as well as energy and spirit. Spirituality is the *experience* of this energy. Spiritual experiences fulfill, animate, enthuse and frighten us. Spirituality is the experience of the sacred and intangible, but an experience with a tangible effect. This energetic aspect essentializes us, it intensifies life but also fear (see "The Story of The Youth Who Went Forth to Learn What Fear Was," a folktale collected by the Brothers Grimm[1]). Whether we like it or not, spirituality is difficult to reconcile with everyday reality. Spirituality is so profoundly attractive, precisely because it leads us to the outermost source of energy and to the *mysterium tremendum et fascinans* ("the fearful and fascinating mystery": Otto 1917/1987).

But where, I wonder, is the sphere of the demons and the demonic? First and last, innermost and outermost, only God or the Whole, the divine, the Being, the light *really and truly* exist. Here, there is no ambivalence. In this innermost, and at the same time outermost sphere of existence, all energy is pure and free of an adversary such as demons. This uttermost energetic reality has to be imagined as a sphere beyond separation and division, without any false connotations. In this sphere, all is still or once again a single, unified Whole. Thus, there can be no mention of energy split-off. Nothing affects this oneness

---

1   Retrieved from www.grimmstories.com/en/grimm_fairy-tales/the_story_of_the_youth_who_went_forth_to_learn_what_fear_was, accessed on 24 January 2016.

negatively, nothing falls out, nothing has—as depicted in the mythological image of the fallen angel—"fallen off."

Yet, just next to this spaceless and timeless Whole, the liminal sphere begins and the laws of ambivalence become effective: light stands beside darkness, distress beside wellbeing. It is precisely here that total darkness and the dangerously demonic are sometimes experienced. The ego is exposed both to darkness and to its fears (see the case study of Peter; see also Chapter 5). Why here, of all places? A normally developed ego would utterly defy these dimensions. In the liminal sphere, however, the ego's powers, together with its defensive functions and differentiating capacity, are diminished. Fears loom large. The necessitous ego feels naked. Consequently, the ego is confronted with unfiltered, uncontrolled, uncensored energy. It experiences scenarios between angels, fairies and demons, between gentle transport and a perilous undertow. When we face the liminal sphere in the midst of life (for instance, in a nightmare, in a spiritual crisis, in a near-psychotic state, or—in theological terms—in temptation), we need a governing ego, a strong personality and often medical, therapeutic and spiritual assistance. Meditation instructions provide guidance and structure, and require discipline. The Desert Fathers knew about this and stressed the importance of inner presence, of restraining instinctual drives, of asceticism, and of self-knowledge and maturation (Grün 2001). Religions and spiritual practice emphasize ritual and sacrament. Both are important in dealing with the liminal sphere and its nature.

The Liminal Sphere as the Site of Spiritual Struggles

Given the laws of the liminal sphere, we can understand the phenomenon of spiritual struggle. The pervasive theme in this respect is power, above all the question "To whom does power, the final power, belong?" Struggle has two main thrusts, as we learn from terminally ill patients:

1. Does power belong to the ego or to God/the divine? This question concerns the struggle of the ego against its fate, ultimately against God/the divine. The central power question is: "I" or God/the divine/the Whole/the Being/self-determination/"Thy will be done." Rebellion, wrestling with God[2] and bouts of anger are important for lengthy periods during suffering and dying. In many cases, however, at some stage this struggle almost seamlessly merges into denial. An inflated estimation of the human self can lead many people to believe that they are in control of their own life and death, a notion meanwhile widely considered to be "acceptable," at least in Switzerland. Manifold observation of deathbed phenomena has taught me that good dying occurs when patients finally reach the stage of acceptance:

George, aged 30, was causing the nurses and his wife serious problems. Although terminally ill, he believed that meditation would cure him. He accepted music therapy, but not psychology. Whenever he spoke, he was first interrupted by nausea, itching, attacks of pain, and restlessness. This distress persisted. George was unable to utter a sentence without suffering attacks. The more he resisted his illness, the more something inside him rebelled against his resistance. There seemed no way of getting him to understand. Eventually, I too became forceful. "George, you have an awful trouble-maker inside you, who we must fight against." He became calmer and replied that this could well be. Then the itching resumed. He scratched himself. "Listen, I am going to declare war on this trouble-maker. Do you agree?" "Yes," he said and vomited. "All you need to do is to say 'Yes.'"—"Alright, but why should I? I'll never say 'Yes' to my illness after all..." The next attack followed. "Please try to agree, just as a body exercise. When you breathe out, say 'Yes' without thinking about things." He accepted my suggestion. His body became peaceful within seconds. I played some music. He fell asleep. His wife stood beside his bed in sheer

---

2   Many non-religious patients also use the the term God to state his inexistence or to wrestle with him.

disbelief, not understanding but understanding nevertheless. We repeated the exercise a while later. It worked every time. As soon as he began pondering his plight and remembered that he did not actually want to die, the attacks resumed. I taught his wife how to guide her husband through this exercise. Together they practiced saying "Yes" and "Yes," day after day, hour after hour—until George breathed out one last time during the exercise and died, uttering an extended and truly affirmative "Yes."

As observers, we can ask whether we witnessed a magical event or a spiritual struggle. Reflecting on what was happening to his patient before, during, and after these body exercises, the doctor treating George remarked that had he not seen what had happened, not to mention the simplicity of the exercise, he would have thought it was magic. It was not magic, however, but rather this patient's struggle to accommodate his ego to the overriding laws and patterns of life and dying.

2. "Good versus evil, angels versus demons": Does power belong to demons and ghosts, or to God/the divine? This second aspect of the fundamental struggle for power does not directly concern the line of battle between God/the divine and humans, but indirectly. The alternative question is: good spirit versus evil spirit, angels versus demons, light versus darkness, and, above all, the one power—God/the one supreme being—versus powers? These struggles should be understood neither as a theological construct nor as an esoteric fantasy, but as the reality "seen" and experienced by individuals, for instance, the dying. So the conclusion that everyone who struggles in their dying process necessarily has problems with acceptance is too simple. Time and again, there are patients who undergo struggle because they seem to have insight into the great spiritual dimensions behind life and death. Not only do they *cross* the liminal sphere, but they also seem to "understand" parts of its nature. The struggle spells both an imposition and an opportunity.

The more end-of-life and spiritual carers themselves comprehend the phenomenon, and the more pragmatically they learn how to deal with spiritual struggle (see Chapter 9), the better for patients. Spiritual care has to know about and to deal with the liminal sphere, its laws on the threshold of consciousness, as well as with phenomena such as the spiritual experience of darkness, struggle, the difficulties of acceptance, and primordial fear (see Appendix, Figures 10a and b; Renz 2015).

Chapter 3

The Hope
for Grace

Hope and grace, while dissimilar, nevertheless complement each other. Hope is the basic human condition and inner openness into which grace enters, either from without or from within, our innermost being. Hope means to spread the wings of our soul, preparing to take flight without knowing whether those wings will carry us. Manès Sperber refers to a bridge that, while not actually existing, forms step-by-step under the feet of those who dare to set foot across the abyss (Hommes 1980: 22).

Hope and Healing are Daring Words

Holger had been suffering from cancer for 20 years and still had many years to live. Persistent nausea and a slowly growing tumor afflicted him: At times he wanted to die, at other times he wanted to live. It was as if a leaden weight hung over Holger and his wife in his hospital room. My first impulse was to run away, to avoid becoming depressed myself. Should I engage with this patient and risk the unknown? Following several long conversations about his inner homelessness, Holger finally agreed to music-assisted relaxation. During the intervention, he grew very quiet and experienced himself as being borne aloft and weightless: "I felt great love; I felt wrapped in a warm, comfortable covering." This was, as I later realized, an initiation experience. From that point, I tried to reach Holger through small signals. But nothing else happened. On returning home after one of our sessions, I suddenly began shaking my head while doing some housework and exclaimed: "This is unbearable!—Isn't this too much for anyone to endure?" No sooner had I uttered my frustration than I noticed a change of attitude, from helplessness and pity to new respect for Holger and his wife. I decided to share this feeling with them the next day. They were moved. My intuition was that at the height of a crisis a creative force bursts forth. Before I could share this thought with Holger and his wife, she said: "You seem different today. Are you feeling hopeful?" "Yes," I replied, although I could not explain why. Hope is irrational, I added. "You know, I just want to hope for something better, whatever it will be." A gentle smile crossed her face, before she began crying and fell silent. Months later, after Holger had spent some time at home, we met again. Neither he nor his wife were much better. And yet they smiled: "We were looking forward to seeing you and we often thought of you...I must have wanted to call you at least a hundred times but never did," Holger explained. The mere thought of our encounters had given them strength, his wife added. Despite the circumstances, a fundamental change had occurred; something had grown, intangibly, over the past months, something like an island of hope. For me, this was a small miracle—grace! Evidently, the above initiation experience was the beginning. A sense of home had arisen amidst the previous homelessness. Home, I now realized, was the seedbed of hope.

Hope or illusion? Hope is a difficult word in an oncology and palliative care unit. What may we hope for if a patient's condition does nothing but deteriorate? Hopelessness must have its place, but so must the longing for hope. Even illusory hope must be permitted. Many patients feel subjectively better amidst (illusory) hope than without any hope at all. Hope is like the driving force, while its actual concretization—"*What may I hope for?*"—gradually alters:

> *From the hope of getting well to the hope*
> *of experiencing good times again.*
> *From the hope of living to the hope of dying well.*
> *From the hope for oneself to a hope beyond oneself.*

Hope concerns the vision of a future yet to come. It is about the expectation of fulfillment and about change.

No less hazardous than the mention of hope within the hospital context is the talk of healing and "salvation." What does this mean? And how, if at all, does "healing" understood thus, occur?

Carola, a young deaf woman (her loss of hearing appeared to be congenital), lay on her deathbed. What struck me was that she responded to my playing of the ocean drum (which recalls the gentle sounds of the sea) with gently rolling movements. Then she asked me to leave her room. I soon discovered more about this woman's tragedy, caught between isolation and a thirst for life, from conversations with her relatives. She was utterly unable to accept death, they told me, and had always aspired to life and beauty. She had always begged for love. At my next visit, Carola lay on her bed, her face tense. Her sister sat beside her, ready to translate my words into sign language. But Carola did not open her eyes anymore. I felt distance. She seemed to be beyond reach. What could I do? Saying nothing was not an option: the tension was too strong, her face too contorted. Finally, I spoke into the void: "Carola, I am speaking to you although you can perhaps not hear me: if you are afraid, do not remain there, but go forth." And some minutes later, I continued, "You will be beautiful in another way." My words prompted deep breathing and sighing. "She has understood you," her sister exclaimed and added, "I love you Carola…you will be beautiful, you may leave now." "Rrrl." Carola slipped away from the here and now, as if entering a terminal state. The next day, after a visit from the chaplain, she died. Like me, her sister was convinced that when approaching death Carola had "heard and understood."

Salvation, as conceived by many religions, needs to be distinguished from wellbeing in a medical sense and also from sheer happiness. Salvation, or being healed, describes that inner state in which we are whole, unscathed, and identical to our essence, irrespective of any external demands or any neurotic inclinations. In the words of D. Sulmasy: "Healing is about the restoration of right relationships" (2006: 125). Adults are normally disconnected from such a state, but yearning for connection, maturation, and spiritual experiences brings them closer. One biblical word for salvation, or healing, is to be blessed. Of all people, the critically ill have taught me that, regardless of suffering, states of blessing and spiritual experiences do in fact exist. Crucially, however, we cannot produce our own salvation: its experience is fragmentary, no more than momentary and granted to us by divine grace. Salvation, then, means a profound form of being-at-one-with-oneself and being with the sacred, with the divine—"with-God." Salvation is the opposite of alienation and narcissistic isolation. Many dying feel disconnected and yearn for salvation.

All of us long for a happy and blessed life. Each biography tells the story of a life between wholeness and disintegration. Deep inside, each spiritual process is driven by the longing for healing, for becoming whole. Therapy seeks to awaken buried intuitions and yearnings, so that these may become the power of hope. Carola's yearning consisted of a longing for beauty and love. What she probably had been deprived of during her life, seemed to happen in approaching death.

The Dark Night: The Modern Person's Experience Versus that of the Mystic

One of the laws of spiritual experience is that they often occur at the nadir of suffering: That is, when our final resistance or struggle gives way to acceptance and exhaustion. Religiously speaking, the experience of God often begins when we reach the impasse of godforsakenness and inner derangement.

Manuela, in her fifties, was a cultivated woman whose zest for life bordered on lust, or even greed. She was determined not to accept her illness. She was suffering under her hardened stance, which deprived her of any joy. She had been coming for therapy at longer intervals for two years. Her anger at God, at her fate and at me was getting worse. One day, I telephoned her at home. For Manuela, who had grown up without genuine motherly love, my call—and the subsequent intervention with music-assisted relaxation—afforded her the experience of a mother, the experience of being without fear or forlornness. In her own terms, it was an experience of God. Soon, however, she was once again filled with anger and distress. She could not understand that the world would go on without her, as if she had never existed. Moreover, she was suffering from physical paralysis, pain, constriction. The next time I entered her room, the air was thick, as if she were already dead. Manuela lisped: "Monika, I can hardly breathe." Her oppressiveness overwhelmed me. After a while, I asked her: "Are you still there?" "Yes." The atmosphere was hardly conducive to dying, "Manuela, we need another ally; it won't work like this." "What do you mean?" "We—I—need God here." "No!" The oppressiveness persisted, as if anger lay suffocated within. At some point, I intervened: "Manuela— for your own sake—we need more substantial help. Do you agree?" "Yes." "You know that running against a brick wall will be in vain. Nor can your anger persist, no matter how understandable it is. I suggest that I send your anger where it belongs—namely, to God—here in the chapel. This is a ritual, but more than that. Please try to express your anger in words and then give it to me." She looked at me sceptically: "Are you sure?" A minute's silence. I was beginning to think that I would have to abandon the exercise—only for Manuela to say unexpectedly: "Okay." Together, word by word, we expressed and felt her anger. "I just don't want to die." "I understand, but do you prefer to suffer like this, without any prospect of improvement?" "Oh..." she sighed deeply. "No—here you are, take my anger."

When I returned the next day, Manuela gave me a warm welcome: "I would never have thought...no sooner had you left the room, the anger was gone... I could breathe and felt free. Nothing mattered anymore—well, not exactly. In fact, everything mattered, as if everything would succeed, and as if there were a greater objective." The atmosphere in the room was now sacred. We remained silent. Finally, I told her about Pierre Teilhard de Chardin (1881–1955) and his mystical vision of being drawn to a goal (Teilhard de Chardin 1955/1959: 256). Moreover, this meant that at death one was not extinguished, but mysteriously integrated into a greater whole and order. She nodded silently and remained relaxed and free of fear for days. Another attack followed later: Everything felt leaden, she said, "far worse than the deepest night." "Yes, it is a feeling of being motherless, of profound abandonment, of a remoteness from God," I added. The silence persisted for quite some time, before the atmosphere relaxed. Manuela said: "Now, I shall just lie here." The tone of her voice suggested acceptance. I expressed my respect. We exchanged glances. Manuela breathed deeply, as if something had been achieved. As she became more and more tired and peaceful, her life slowly faded away.

To endure such an impasse and nadir of suffering is one of the hardest challenges for patients and spiritual caregivers. It seems as if time stands still. Complete and utter hopelessness—physical, psychological, spiritual—descends. Besides the actual illness and an all-encompassing sense of powerlessness, a secondary affliction emerges: an emphatic sense of existential degradation (Sölle 1993: 96–7, 173). A once forceful and sometimes vain ego is now subdued, in effect "dead." We are no more than a creature and feel no longer "human." We seem deprived of any sense of happiness, performance and meaningfulness. Indeed, we even lack the strength to endure the coming hour. Our only option at this juncture is capitulation. God, too, is far away, uninvolved, not almighty but powerless, or even nonexistent. Grace, as a bridge to heaven or to a higher power, is missing. The darkness inside us is eerily soundless, leaden, hollow. All we can do is to "hold on," even if this means little else than daring to take the next breath. Thus, holding on is a "decision" we take. This decision is not willed, but "lived and breathed" and, as such, an act of final loyalty. Finding an attitude of acceptance, verbally or nonverbally, has to be done by ourselves.

What happens positively amidst suffering, however, is not limited to spiritual experience and grace. What we endure helps our whole personality to grow. We are less and less merely victims of our human predicament, or determined defencelessly by our suffering, but are able to adopt an inner stance toward our suffering (I have discussed the experience of dignity elsewhere; see Renz 2015). Here, we grow more mature and dignity emerges, and in both move beyond the limitations our creatureliness.

What distinguishes our modern experience from what mystics like John of the Cross (1542–1591) called "the dark night of the soul?"[1] For Christian mystics like him, the *unio mystica* and the "dark night," the experience of God and the "experience of nonexperience," belong together. The experience of the night comprises the uttermost experience of longing. At the nadir of God's absence, he is nevertheless present, albeit

---

1   "Where have you hidden, *Beloved*, and left me moaning? You fled like the *stag* After wounding me; I went out calling you, and you were gone," John of the Cross (transl. 1987: 221).

negatively. While this leads us to mention the mystical night of love and the nocturnal remoteness from God in the same breath, we have no sense of how abyssmally and how infinitely long the impasse and the despair lying inbetween can last. We must beware not to mystically overinflate this impasse too rashly. There has to be an interval of emptiness, as happens with Holy Saturday between Good Friday and Easter Day, for instance. Mystics and saints of various religions were also familiar with the dark, unfathomable precipices of human existence. However, a mystic's experience differs from the nights suffered by most desperate patients nowadays. What distinguishes mystics and saints is their inner connection with God/the divine or their seemingly repeated experience of that connection. Somehow and at some stage, the mystic has made a fundamental decision: namely, to say "Yes" to God, to a supreme being, although he suffers tremendous distress and forsakenness. He is guided by what we might call the longing for love, by an inner teacher, by inner strength, maybe by Christ. The mystic carries within him an island of spirituality, from which he dares to leap into the dark void, time after time.

Today, many people in our civilization, do not—or no longer—have this inner place of refuge. We are unpracticed in the spiritual path through darkness. Sudbrack (1999: 29) observed: "Can 'I' endure the 'negative myticism' of suffering and darkness if the existential basis, a 'positive experience' of basic trust in God/the divine, and feeling secure with him, is missing?" In our study at the oncology and palliative care units of St. Gallen Cantonal Hospital, only very few patients endured the inner darkness on their own. All others first almost despair. All the more important therefore is therapeutic and spiritual support. It is not until afterwards that we realize that God/the divine had already been present during our impasse (as theology puts it), suffering with us but just as powerless.

Lending Hope

End-of-life and spiritual caregivers are not healers, they are indeed intermediaries. Besides empathically accompanying patients, in some cases caregivers may grasp, either consciously or representatively, what stands unconsciously in the way of the ill. As caregivers, we lend patients our spiritual strength, sometimes even our dreams. We sometimes compassionately endure our patients' tension and hopelessness up to the point when something constellates itself in their innermost being: the felicitous word or a beneficial impulse. Sometimes, the helpful impulse first emerges in our own heart and mind.

The fact that at some point transformation and grace will happen is inherent in any approach to psychotherapy and spiritual care. Both follow the inner guidance that emerges from within the patient. Both try to share the actual darkness of patients. Creative solutions arise precisely from consciously enduring tension, whether this involves an inner spiritual struggle, an existential fear amidst our illness or difficult family dynamics.

> *One evening, I was standing at the bedside of Anita, an about 50-year-old dying mother of two. Anita suffered from terrible pain, nauseating swellings, a deep fear of suffocation, and a despair that had almost developed a life of its own. Relaxation proved impossible! I tried various things. Words that had offered support in the past failed to reach her now. She grew calm for about three minutes when I left my telephone number on her bedside table so that she could call me that night. A brief glimmer of joy crossed her face, followed by more despair. "Anita, it's not about having the strength for the next few days, but for the next few minutes, for the next breath. I would like to endure as much of your pain with you as possible. You matter to me, I'm not indifferent to your plight." A ray of hope, then again despair. We persevered until well into the evening.*

All of a sudden, I exclaimed: "Anita, every minute longer that you endure is a blessing for Natalie and Karin (her adolescent daughters, who she was worried about)." Anita breathed and slowly relaxed. The atmosphere had changed and had given rise to something new: hope. She said that I could leave now. Three days later, more relaxed and suffering less pain, she told me: "It was so important that I didn't die that night. That would have been a terrible death for my family." What I had said about her children had helped her survive that night. And she could breathe. The power of motherly love had pierced the emotional numbness caused by her fear of death.

My experience with Anita that night took effect. The next day, I had arranged to meet Dorothee Sölle (1929–2009), the German liberation theologian. I was still under the influence of the encounter I had had the night before. I recounted the events in Anita's room. Dorothee was impressed, in particular, about how Anita and I had found a way out of her despair and helplessness to reach a turning point. Dorothee and I then shared other experiences, before she suddenly interrupted me: "What you just mentioned, that Anita's perseverance would come as a blessing for her children, isn't really acceptable, you know. You could never have kept that promise." Without a second thought, I replied: "But precisely, that is my task, *to keep reaching a state of hope* (however one formulates it). In Anita's case, for instance, my hope was that at least some of her personality and radiance would reach her children. The problem, though, is to keep achieving hope. I face this challenge every week, often even several times a day. It takes great self-discipline, and I need to overcome my reluctance and spiritual resistance if I am to help patients." My words caught Dorothee's interest. We agreed that there must be a connection between a closeness to reality, without any mystical overinflation, and an attitude of hope. Hope, we realized, is a state of being, not of having…and if we manage to be hopeful, the strength, radiance, and persuasiveness of faith will simply emerge. Presumably, such being is now the exception rather than the rule. *Reaching* hope is a continual challenge and grace.

"It is impossible to find sufficient hope just in ourselves"

These were the words of the German political theologian Johann Baptist Metz (b. 1928) (Metz 1975: 99).

A recent report on development assistance notes that the Salesians of Don Bosco founded a village in Columbia to look after destitute street children and former child soldiers (girls and boys aged 14 to 19). A team of educators, therapists, craftspersons, and spiritual caregivers helps the children to reintegrate into the human community, step by step. Apprenticeship workshops provide skills training aimed at ensuring that the children have a professional future. The former child soldiers, who have fallen out of the network of human relationships, present the most formidable challenge. Crucial progress occurs when the children once again meet one or several members of their own family who are brought to the village often from far away. The reunion is accompanied by a blessing ceremony. After this day, the educators and caregivers feel the attempts at reintegration will succeed.

Whose future could be more dismal than that of a child soldier? What might offer hope under such circumstances? The example of the Salesian Society suggests that hope springs from the prospect of human community, the feeling of belonging and subsequent reintegration. And yet this alone is not enough. A flame must be reignited in an extinguished soul, for instance, through an encounter with the long lost mother, father, a brother, or a sister.

Johann Baptist Metz replied, when asked what the Church was, that "no one can have enough hope on their own." The "Church" and Christianity, he argued, should be imagined as a community of hope (1 Peter 3.15) that conveys an atmosphere of familiarity grounded in God/the divine. As bearers of hope, communities function for the individual as a therapeutic relationship does. Whereas we cannot coax each other into hope, an intimate or a religious bond or community provides a feeling of belonging and shared existence, and perseverance. However, the feeling of hope comes as a gift of grace alone (*sola gratia*).

Chapter 4

Experience of Transcendence as Reality and Grace

Experiences of Transcendence and their Effects

Spiritual experiences of transcendence are real, even common, amidst suffering (see Renz *et al.* 2015). In our study, no fewer than 135 of the 251 patients surveyed had *one or several such experiences* (see Appendix, Figure 1; see also Arnold and Lloyd 2013; Fenwick, Lovelace and Brayne 2010). This frequency is astonishing—and yet on the other hand it is not: experiences of transcendence occur more frequently near death, but also during incisive crisis, serious illness and convalescence (see Chapter 2).

In addition, experiences of transcendence have a profound impact. Sometimes, such experiences are obvious or veiled announcements of approaching death. Post-death observations made by the families and friends of the deceased typically attest: "He said so," "She could see it coming," and "He obviously knew it was about to happen." Spiritual experiences seem to facilitate the dying process (Fenwick and Brayne 2011; Kerr *et al.* 2014). In our study, 30 out of 135 patients with spiritual experiences died within a few minutes after having such an experience or within the hour (!); three patients died in the midst of such an experience (see Appendix, Figure 2). Whether in life or before death, experiences of transcendence have lasting effects: they intensify the quality of existence, establish identity, and initiate a new attitude toward life. We observed that all 135 patients experienced better body awareness and an altered sense of the "here and now." The altered awareness of space, time and one's body appears to be characteristic of spiritual experience—similar states are reported in near-death experiences; experts use the term "nonlocal awareness" (see Lommel 2010; Fenwick 2010). In our study, about half of the patients reported considerable pain relief (71) and less anxiety (75).[1] Equally, about half our patients expressed a changing attitude toward life and death (71), toward their illness (71) and toward God/the divine (68; see Appendix, Figure 3). Similar effects may also occur in the midst of life, triggered, for instance, by a profound dream or by music-assisted active imagination.

Our project revealed that the effects of experiences of transcendence can be measured not only in terms of facts and figures. Every change, even the slightest shift, was felt to be a gift. Effects included, for instance, a new sensuousness, a capacity for love, inner freedom, identity, and dignity. Here are some examples:

Ismael, a 40-year-old Albanian man, who was mature, self-confident and devout at the same time, was ashamed of the misdemeanors of his countrymen, but still leaped to their

---

1   A particular nuance is worth noting in this respect: Contrary to a person's spiritual *attitude*, which according to King *et al.* (2013) does not reduce anxiety, spiritual *experiences* significantly relieve fear regardless of a person's religious or spiritual attitude. The explanation would seem to be that attitudes are largely ego-determined, whereas experiences of transcendence, because they cannot be produced by the ego, are all the more powerful.

defence: "Honestly, Monika, Muslims are not evil. Muslims are deeply religious, I swear." Did I have any reason not to believe him, I ventured? This question made him deeply thoughtful. Once he had considered matters, our relationship was like a done deal. Furthermore, we were allies. Ismael accepted me, a Christian, in terms of his code of honor. Also, he felt that I recognized his efforts to bridge the cultural divide between our religions. "Ismael," I assured him on one occasion, "individuals like you are important." "What?! Say that again. Do you really think so?" He wept for hours. His pain had lessened. Although I had done nothing in particular, his depression lifted for many weeks. In future, he told me, he wanted us to pray to Allah and to God as one. Later, his mistrust was back, and he struggled against it. Then, he observed: "What you said at the time was a sacred oath." The fact that I believed in him had evidently given Ismael the space and self-esteem to recognize himself as a person in his own right.

Mariette remained standing in the doorway, trembling with fear. She didn't want any "primal scream therapy, no drumming, nothing pious." Before me stood a mature but deeply fearful woman, who soon began to trust me and told me her life story: she had been hurt all her life, ever since early childhood! She had constantly felt out of place. She was afraid before going to the doctor's. "I would also be afraid if I were you," I observed. "What? But then I'm quite normal." "Yes, of course you are." I then told Mariette about the spiritual experiences one of my patients was having: she had received protection from a guardian angel, who had been present even during the doctor's examination. This aroused Mariette's interest. Her fear disappeared completely during music-assisted active imagination. "There was a desert—a wide expanse— freedom." She had not experienced this before. Vastness contrasts with narrowness, which is closely related to fear. I asked Mariette whether freedom was stronger than fear. "Oh, yes, there is no fear where this freedom is." In three subsequent music-assisted relaxations, Mariette's desert became an oasis. Instead of constant fear, she now experienced sensuousness and a connection with the "hear and now." "I feel so damned good," she told me. "For years, others lived my life; now I am alive, living it myself. I now enjoy sitting on my balcony, eating raspberries and looking at flowers. And, during the examination at my doctor's, your voice was so present, telling me that I am normal." Several months later, Mariette was readmitted to hospital. Once again, she had desert and oasis experiences. A capacity for love emerged from within her that could not have been greater. She could give everything to others, including herself. She praised everyone. And what about her fear? "No, I'm not afraid. Dying is freedom."

Noah, a leukemia patient, had been suffering from phobias for years. His life felt like a prison, he told me. He felt unable to leave home without a compelling reason, ever since his cat had died. He was not able to go out for walks. When he opened the window, he saw bars in front of it. Although he knew that this was sheer fantasy, he still could not imagine the window without bars. What had he done professionally? A long time ago, he told me, he had lost his job as an accountant. He had then founded a consulting firm using a fictitious customer file. His business was flourishing, but he had no clients. What did he live on? "I don't really know, a pension." I felt close to tears. Noah then mentioned that he had sought out my help for another reason: he had dreamed that he would be healthy and free once more, which was why he wanted to try therapy again. Healthy? Leukemia was not a problem compared to the mental burden. I barely knew what to say. "It is terrible to live like this; it is exhausting," I said. And I could only admire him for keeping reality and fantasy apart, and that he had lived in this prison for so long. "That is a tremendous achievement." "What do you mean?" Noah was taken aback. Did I believe he had a chance of recovery? "It is a long path...but you must believe your dreams." "What?" He felt comforted, he told me.

He contacted me a week later. Our session had helped. His body felt different, no longer like a prison, but simply ill: "And there are holes in the bars." He had again dreamed that he would recover and be released from prison. I was impressed. But I did not dare interpret Noah's dream. What did recovery mean, let alone freedom? We bid farewell. A week later, he died, unexpectedly.

Onah, a patient in his early fifties, lay on his bed, radiant and accepting things as they were—for weeks! He loved orthodox choral music, but most of all silence. What, I wondered, was the secret of his radiance? Was he religious? The Bible was always with him and he prayed to God, simply repeating the words "God, God." What I sensed bordered on a form of love mysticism between God/the divine and us humans.

Hans-Rudolf, whose life had been interrupted abruptly by illness, told me that he had no religious affiliation, that he was disappointed with God and that he was actually an atheist. Yet he called the music that I played for him "spiritual." Apart from that he was quite erratic, jumping from one subject to another: Why, he wondered, did he sweat so profusely? Other patients sweated out of fear, I replied, but that did not seem to be his problem. "No!" he exclaimed brusquely. I sensed a power struggle, a stifling of issues and feelings, and cautiously asked Hans-Rudolf: "Are you consternated because you have been torn out of your life so suddenly? I would also feel angry." He nodded nonchalantly. "Could it be that you haven't come to terms with fate yet?" "Yes, could be." The atmosphere in the room was tense. He sweated even more. "Don't you sometimes feel angry, for instance, at God?" I said "Yes, of course I do" he replied. "I sometimes hear myself saying, 'God, that's enough now!' But then nothing happens anyway." I ask "Could you imagine us trying to settle your 'account' with fate, so that I say an informal prayer and place your 'account,' your anger, your distress before God?" "No!" Despite his refusal, Hans-Rudolf wanted me to stay. We talked about various topics, until he suddenly ordered me to pray. Utterly taken by surprise, I listened to myself and began: "God, whoever or whatever you are, before you lies Hans-Rudolf, in great distress and in terrible suffering."—"Don't say 'Hans-Rudolf' when you pray. That sounds too arrogant. I am no more than a worm anyway," he interrupted me and began weeping. I was at a loss for words, but then managed to say: "For me, you are not simply a worm before God. May I say in my prayer, 'Here lies Hans-Rudolf?'" "Yes, please try!" During my prayer, he became devout, then said: "Yes, 'Hans-Rudolf' sounds right." He was still crying. A man previously on his guard had now become someone who had had a profound experience. From this moment on, there was no more sweating, no restlessness, no gruffness, but instead kindness. Contrary to expectation, Hans-Rudolf died within a few days. During his last breaths, he stammered that the "experience" had made the difference.

Do Experiences of Transcendence Depend on a Religious Attitude?

We found that religious identity grows with experiences of transcendence. Sixty-eight out of the 135 patients who had spiritual experiences reported a new attitude toward God/ the divine. All 68 patients, who included 9 atheists/agnostics, either used the term "God" at least once or had an "Aha" moment, namely, that HE or IT or a gift of grace had been involved. Thus, spiritual experiences are not reserved for religious persons (see Appendix, Figures 5 and 6). On the contrary, the 135 patients reporting one or several spiritual experiences were people with various religious attitudes and from different religious backgrounds, including 20 atheists/ agnostics (see Appendix, Figure 6).[2]

2 According to Sulmasy, each person is a being "in relationship with the transcendent—even if by way of rejecting the very possibility of transcendence" and even atheists are thus "intrinsically spiritual" (Sulmasy 2006: 14).

Nevertheless, the factor of religion is far from negligible as regards spiritual experience. Many people consider religious longing, an orientation toward God, a relationship with sacred texts, sacraments, church interiors and religious songs to be a gateway to spiritual experience (in our project, 85 patients, affiliated or unaffiliated to a religious community, including the Christian, agnostic, Muslim, and some other communities, reported such access to their spiritual experience at least once; among these 85 patients were also 49 who experienced a "wrestling with God" (see Renz *et al.* 2015; Appendix, Figure 9).

Do earlier spiritual experiences (within the context of near-death experience, religious faith, meditation, a spiritual crisis or psychosis) open the door to other experiences of the transcendent? Our project answers this question in various ways: the 135 patients reporting spiritual experiences included many *with* earlier experiences of the transcendent, but also others who, because of their previous life, *had never given the matter any thought*, let alone dared to consider themselves capable of such experience (see Appendix, Figure 7). Among these last mentioned patients were a mathematician, a foreman and a business administration specialist. Potentially, I argue, we are all capable of spiritual experience.

However, our findings suggest that any kind of fixation stands in the way of spiritual experience. Fixation in general prevents us from experiencing something unexpected. Concerning religious attitudes, fixation manifests itself in an adherence to dogmatic religious belief, as well as in embittered anti-religiousness. The meditation master who believed that his spiritual power would help him to heal himself of cancer also suffered from a fixation. We must let go of such fixations *first of all*.

Ulrich, a member of a strict free church, was convinced that his sins would overpower him after his death and obstruct his passage to rebirth. And yet he did not want to be reborn according to the teachings of his church. For days, he lay on his bed, his limbs stiff, his body weary, his face rigid and hollowed. But he had no doubts and his concept of God remained unchanged. Music touched him at times, but not at others. One morning though, he saw figures in his room, and after a blessing, anger surfaced, followed by profuse sweating. Everyone was relieved. The next morning, he told me that the figures were still present but had changed. They were now luminous. Guilt was no longer an issue, only "light." He died peacefully that evening.

Reality Testing: How Do I Know that I have had a Spiritual Experience?

Both experts and non-specialists ask me time and again how we can recognize spiritual experience. How can we distinguish the spiritual from the profane? How do we know whether something spiritual has occurred or not?

In the final instance, any precise knowledge remains elusive. This skepticism, however, keeps us attentive, and for that very reason I am grateful for a questioning attitude. Experiences are intimate and individual: each of us has our own truth, in which there are no absolute guidelines, no right or wrong answers. Even our interpretations of ourselves are no more than interpretations and therefore no more than a limited (that is, partial) truth. Interpretations can be distortions, caused by unconscious fear, projections, and formative influences. Each culture impresses its particular stamp on its adherents, and thus interpretations are culturally (pre)determined. The same dream motif (for instance, an elephant, a rose, a snow-clad landscape, a vast ocean) has a different meaning if dreamed by an Indian or by a Swiss person. Even more care is needed when interpreting spiritual experiences because phenomenologically every such experience remains to some extent elusive, blurred and inaccessible to our ego's scrutiny.

Our project took several precautionary measures to distinguish the spiritual from the profane. Only those spiritual experiences were recorded that both patient *and* therapist recognized or at least nonverbally affirmed as spiritual. Possible visible effects (total peace, deliverance from fear) provided evidence of spiritual experience beyond a patient's verbal account. Such effects facilitated the recognition of spiritual experience. Whenever the patient or therapist doubted the spiritual nature of an experience, or whenever patients affirmed the sacred character of their experience only inadequately, that experience was excluded from evaluation. The experiences of confused patients were also excluded in consultation with the responsible physicians and caregivers. Patients diagnosed with schizophrenia or psychosis were excluded from the survey from the outset.

How were spiritual experiences communicated? In most cases, communication was spontaneous. Fifty-nine patients conveyed *all* of their spiritual experiences of their own accord and thus spontaneously. Forty-seven patients reported at least *one* of their spiritual experiences while talking about themselves; in these cases, my questions helped patients to discover the moving nature of their experience and to construe the spiritual character of the impression it made on them. Twenty-nine patients could no longer form complete sentences or were deeply affected by such experience at least *once*. However, they unmistakably affirmed, either by stammering or nodding, the sacred nature of their experience and its possible effects (see Appendix, Figure 8).

Our cautious approach leads me to assume that *other* patients also had experiences of transcendence. These patients, however, were not recorded, either because they were unable or too shy to share their experiences (on such limitations, see Renz *et al.* 2015). Thus, we are dealing with *minimum* figures, which merit even greater attention. However, neither the frequency nor the visible effects of experiences of the transcendent prove that such experience is an expression of grace. Unverifiability is intrinsic to grace.

Can Experiences of Transcendence be Triggered?

"What favors spiritual experience?" I am often asked this question, in the compelling hope that such experience can be worked toward. However, no matter how impressive spiritual experiences and their effects may be, they cannot be educed or "elicited." In a preliminary phase of our project, we realized beyond doubt that as long as we expected and focused on spiritual experiences, they failed to occur. This was true even when patients sought to produce such experience themselves. No experience occurred in such cases, leaving patients irritated, often to the point of frustration. We therefore abandoned any kind of focus and instead relied on observation (see the methodology discussion in the Introduction). Transcendence, as the old German folktale of Mother Hulda suggests, is not readily "available": despite her cunning, Pechmarie (Pitch-Mary) cannot retrieve the gold given to Goldmarie (Gold-Mary) in the underworld.[3] Gold is not money—and unlike money it cannot be minted at will.

Phenomenological research can, in contrast, record and evaluate the observable circumstances accompanying spiritual experiences. Key questions in this respect include: What

---

3   In this folktale, a girl sits at a spinning wheel and spins all day until she hurts her finger and the spindle gets bloody. She wants to wash the spindle, but it falls into the well. Her stepmother demands her to jump down the well to fetch the spindle. She finds herself on a meadow, full of sunshine and beautiful flowers. She comes to an oven full of baked bread, to a tree full of ripe apples, and to the little house of the great Mother Hulda (an archetypal mother). There she does the housework and gets enough good food. After a longer or shorter time in the underworld, which is beyond time and space, she gets homesick even if she has a better life in the underworld. Mother Hulda guides her back to the gate to the upper world and gives her back the spindle and lots of gold. Her sister also wants to have the gold but is insensitive to the underworld and its rules. Standing under the gate, the sister isn't showered with gold but covered with sticky pitch. The two girls are called Gold Mary and Pitch Mary. See "Mother Hulda," Grimms' Fairy Tales, retrieved from www.grimmstories.com/en/grimm_fairy-tales/mother_hulda (accessed February 2, 2015).

immediately preceded a spiritual experience (for instance, a therapeutic intervention, a conversation about religion, etc.)? What were the accompanying circumstances? What did patients subsequently associate with the experience? Our evaluation of such accompanying circumstances confirmed the importance of music-assisted active imagination, relaxation, religious support (including the wrestling with God), empathy, dreams, and maturation processes (see Appendix, Figure 9). Whereas the question about the limiting or explanatory links between experiences of transcendence and medication must be raised, it cannot be answered conclusively.[4]

The Various Forms of Experiences of Transcendence

Experiences of transcendence occur in various forms, either magnificently or subtly, typically in the form of either simple experience, creative activity, or inspiration and recognition. In any case, such experiences represent a breakthrough.

Extraordinary experiences

It is widely believed that peak experiences (Maslow 1962/1994) occur even if we have the impression that they only happen

---

4   One limitation of our project is that we do not fully understand the effect of medication on the spiritual experiences of palliative-care patients (see Renz *et al.* 2015). On the one hand, terminally ill patients naturally shift between different states of consciousness, *with*, *despite*, or *irrespective* of medication. For this reason, neither a patient's states of mind nor the reasons for these states are always entirely clear. Medication was administered consistently on *medical* grounds and according to the *physical* needs of patients, and never due to particular project-related interests. The experiences of confused or psychotic patients were not recorded. Without doubt, medication and a change of consciousness are linked (see Grof 1985/1991). Whether a change of consciousness can be equated with spiritual experience, however, remains a matter of interpretation. Patient accounts repeatedly suggest that spiritual experiences coincide with an expansion of consciousness, but such experience reaches even further.

to other people. Such magnificent experiences enter our lives forcefully or imploringly. The individual feels compelled to deepen or reorient (that is, change) his or her identity and lifestyle. In the midst of a severe illness, such extraordinary experiences sometimes correspond to and coincide with an unforeseeable turn in the course of illness:

> *Sonia, a woman of about 50 years of age, raised as a Protestant, was terrified of the dark, until she noticed that her fear was similar to that she had suffered in a coma after a car accident as a young woman. She remembered that she had felt terribly cold. She wept. I asked: had there been nothing beautiful that had given her protection? She fell silent. She had never really spoken about the following experience: "It was as if a bearded man were standing on the left side of my bed. I was actually paralyzed. The man said: 'Peace be with you. You will rise again.' He gave me courage." A few months later, defying medical prognosis, Sonia had managed to get out of bed and walk again and make a full recovery. Years later, she had recognized the man in a television documentary: Padre Pio. She had taken no interest in God or religion before her experience, let alone in saints. "But—it was him." She wept. I was impressed. Together, we managed to relate her former experience to her present fear. This helped her to believe that she was being guided through her new predicament and to feel deeply protected. Her fear of the dark night had since vanished. A week later, Sonia, her face pale, told me: "Padre Pio has visited me again. He told me that the time to die had come." At the end of his visit, she had felt consolation and warmth. I asked her whether she could accept the padre's message? "It's difficult, but yes I can." Two weeks later, she passed away in her sleep.*

Subtle experiences

Spiritual experience also occurs in daily life, in the sensuous simplicity of breathing, in love, in suffering, in affirmations of the present moment, in maturation, and in aging (Rotzetter 2000; Rahner 2004; Nouwen 1992/2007; Rohr 2009). This lends the everyday life of patients a particular intensity: they gaze dreamily up into the crown of a tree; a small joy becomes a great happiness. Even if their concerns and worries are inevitable, even if they are turned over in one's mind, and included in one's prayers—suddenly, at some unexpected turning point, a new perspective emerges and patients relax. Here, then, something divine or holy is at work in its own particular way. Spirituality is actively missed and mercifully found—and without any great fuss! The silent call amid such subtly experienced spirituality is imperative in its own way.

Inspiration, recognition, and creativity as spiritual experience

Deeply spiritual experience also occurs during inspiration. Inspirations determine to a great measure our ability to suddenly to find a solution to a conflict, to achieve a breakthrough in a creative process or to gain insight into something otherwise unkown and unimaginable. Inspirations emerge "out of the blue." Breakthroughs are never produced by the ego, but simply happen. Grace becomes more evident when preceded by struggle, darkness and despair. Many sudden insights and many steps taken toward greater awareness that have shaped world and cultural history, science and research, have sprung from inspiration. Likewise, those "Aha" moments that help us to understand and contextualize our life in new ways are part of spiritual experience.

> *It took her husband's death for one woman to understand how his childhood had overshadowed not only him but also their marriage. Her understanding enabled her to accept her suffering in a new way. She made peace with her dying husband, with her fate including the suffering she had endured with him for years, and with God. And she experienced mercy.*

Where do such breakthroughs and bursts of energy come from? Jungian psychology attributes such movements to the psyche's transcendent function, which according to Erich Neumann causes "a creative third to be born from conflict..." (1960, 358). Theology speaks of the spirit, from life born of the Holy Spirit. This is the factor of grace in the equation.

Can the Contents of Experience be Categorized?

How do patients describe their experiences of transcendence? What exactly does such an experience consist of? Can one distinguish particular categories? These questions were put to me by a senior principal doctor. He asked for an explanatory framework for such occurrences. I shook my head. Categorization, however, was emerging gradually in our project.

Working with patients, we are always first and foremost committed to human welfare. Whether we are a physician, chaplain or spiritual caregiver, therapist or nurse, we listen to patients and respond to their individual needs intuitively. What do they experience? What do they need from us at any given moment (further inquiry, empathy, touch, silence)? Whenever the impression of an experience of transcendence arises, it is important for our counterpart to share this impression. In our project, detailed notes on these experiences were taken. In a second step these journals were analyzed and carefully considered by two independent researchers. Did some kind of order or even a systematics emerge from our analysis? Committed to phenomenological observation as it was, our inquiry focused on *correspondences* (such as the same dream motif, the same status descriptions) and *distinctions*. We soon recognized a difference between an actual experience of Being/God/Wholeness and the experience of marginal phenomena such as angels, a sacred atmosphere and darkness. Numerous experiences contained both aspects. What astonished us when we tallied the 101 accounts that referred to more than merely marginal phenomena. All these patients were touched by the mystery itself (God, the divine, magnificence, the Whole, a supreme being; see Appendix, Table 1 and Figure 3). Sixty-eight patients mentioned the name "God" at least once.

These explicit experiences of Being/God/Wholeness brought forth also the category distinction between the experiences of the One (that is, of unity or Wholeness) and the experiences of an Other (that is, a relationship with an opposite or "Thou," no matter how this was intuited). Experiences of *oneness* such as a wonderful cosmic being stood beside experiences of a *final relationship*, such as honoring and dignity. However, not even these two categories were enough to classify all recorded patient accounts. Where, for instance, did the experience of a red force field belong? What about the experience of a great, protective hand that dissolved more and more into light? Mixed phenomena, and shifts within one and the same experience, were both common.

What ultimately emerged was a categorization into *five central* and *two peripheral* modes of divine experience. The central modes included all aspects of the triune God, but also other configurations of a higher power. Thus, not only the experiences of Christians and members of other religions, but also those of non-religious persons, proved decisive. Categories were determined neither by faith nor by particular concepts of God, but by phenomenology. In *Grenzerfahrung* (2003/2010), my earlier book on this subject, I emphasized only the *five central modes of experience of the transcendent*. Recent experience has taught me that the two types of peripheral experience—of angels and a sacred atmosphere on the one hand, and of darkness and forlornness on the other—are also important. This insight lead me to posit *seven categories* in total (see Appendix, Table 1). These categories help us to interpret experiences of the transcendent in general (of the critically ill, and of healthy persons, for instance, seminar participants).

These seven types of experience are at the heart of this book and are explained in the next two chapters.

Chapter 5

Experiences of Angels and Darkness

Angels and Sacred Atmospheres

Patients in their spiritual experiences of God, of a supreme being, of the holy, but also of angels and the dark night are like modern-day—silent—mystics. In the following two chapters, we shall "listen" to their many experiences.

Angels are messengers in the *liminal sphere* between God/a supreme being on the one hand, and humans on the other, in a preliminary stage of the sacred. They convey messages, such as the one in one woman's dream in which she saw no more than an oversized arm holding out a white gilt-edged envelope toward her. The appearance of an angel or of a luminous figure is *itself* already a message: such spiritual beings announce that God/the divine, is approaching us, even if he or it remains invisible. Angel experiences are often a bridge to the experience of God/the divine (in Elias's dream in Chapter 2, angels appeared as a "preliminary stage" of divine experience). Sometimes, the dying dream of deceased family members who come for them (Fenwick and Brayne 2011), or offer them protection in their distress or send them back into the world of the living. Some patients are touched by the moment of encounter with an angel, others by the holy atmosphere or the vibrational dimension (the flapping wings of an angel).

One patient dreamed of an encounter with his deceased janitor. Contrary to his former everyday life, the janitor now appeared in elegant clothing, wearing other glasses, as a truly charismatic yet faceless figure. He said that he would look after the house and garden.

One dying patient dreamed of an infinitely beautiful room in which an angel had shone forth, like an indirect light, without blinding her. What a magnificent blue!

Another patient saw a sacred room filled with incense. She knew intuitively that here one could be oneself.

Sometimes, angel experiences go hand in hand with a change in the course of an illness, which leaves a particularly deep impression.

Britta, an atheist and a single mother of two boys, suffered from paralysis and impaired vision caused by brain metastases. After lengthy discussions, it was decided to operate. The operation was highly successful: whereas the primary tumor still existed, the paralysis and impaired vision had gone. "It's a miracle," Britta said to me. Immediately after the operation her deceased daughter appeared to her. "She came inside me here," said Britta, pointing to her heart. "Seraina told me not to be sad; I would have some more time to find a godfather for her brothers. And now I feel so well that I can return home next week—That was HIM." Britta wept for hours.

Sometimes, angels take up the struggle against sheer evil, or their light shines forth amidst the menacing darkness.

Darkness, Struggle, Forlornness and Total Threat

What makes our experience of the peripheral spheres of the divine (near-death, awakening from a coma or anaesthetic, nightmares, crises) so difficult? A first, preliminary answer to this question is that this difficulty is characteristic of the "liminal sphere," where the weakened ego experiences itself as miserable, as unprotected, and as godforsaken (see Chapter 2). Experiences of inner and outer darkness are a phenomenon of the liminal sphere, for instance, at the end of life or in traumatic passages in near-death experiences. They have two main characteristics:

One aspect is forlornness, experienced, for instance, as an ice-hole, a glacial cave, or an immeasurable desert.

> *Daniela, a patient about 60 years old, had been traumatized ever since her coma during a previous stay in the intensive-care unit. She allowed no one near her, but she remembered me: "Yes, this woman played music to me in the intensive care unit." She told me about her experience: "I was freezing all the time, as if I were trapped in an ice-hole." She had been trapped for several weeks, my quick mental calculation told me, and I was deeply moved. "May I touch your hands, and tell you in this way that now there is warmth?" She wept and found my touching her wonderful. Then she remembered that at the time the atmosphere had been beautiful before disaster had struck: "I felt well, only to be pushed back into a cold place nearby, a place that felt like a glacial cave." She sobbed and did not stop until I played my small harp: "That is how you played to me in the intensive care unit. It's beautiful." Over several months, Daniela had a profound need to be understood and to understand herself for the first time, and consequently to be consoled.*

A second aspect of experiences of darkness is the opposite of forlornness, namely, total menace (eerie darkness, roaring sounds, "devouring" or steamrolling machinery, giant wild animals and so on). Both aspects are a frequent peripheral experience of the sacred. It indicates that we have moved dangerously close to the numinous.

An elderly woman had a dream of a steamrolling machinery at the entrance of a large cave. She had to pass this entrance. She pushed a tin can under the machinery and got a shock from seeing how the machinery crushed the can. "That could happen to me as well," she thought. She shrank and shrank until she was tiny enough to enter the cave. The scenery of the machinery had now disappeard and before here opened a sacred room filled with incense. (See also Peter and Elias in Chapter 2.)

These two aspects of dark experiences are identical to the two aspects of primordial fear that I have introduced elsewhere (Renz 2015). Going through this dark night prepares the ego for an encounter with the sacred. It evokes feelings of one's own creatureliness and dependence. Patients are reminded that power belongs not to the ego but to the absolute, to a supreme being, called God or otherwise (see Chapter 2—the first aspect of primardial fear concerns the problem of the ego versus a higher power/a supreme being/God).

A second answer to the question about what makes our experience of the liminal spheres so difficult refers to a power struggle between good and evil. This second experience of the dark lets humans participate in this major spiritual struggle: "God versus evil, light versus darkness, angels versus demons (see Chapter 2, second question). This second kind of struggle also includes experiences of "the devil," "witches and being tormented," curses versus blessings, or ghost scenarios:

A dying woman aged 40 told me the following dream: "I was living in a ruined city around 300 BCE I don't understand this dream, but it was telling me: the city is full of evil, living amidst the ruins and grabbing hold of me."

In the middle of a panic attack, a terminally ill patient pointed at her husband and screamed: "The devil." I knew the husband and said spontaneously: "No, that it isn't the devil. But there seems to be a devil in the room. Do you need to be protected?" "Yes, please!" I drew the sign of the cross on the woman's hand, forehead, and body...and opened the window. She grew calmer and said: "Now the air is clean." A while later, her spiritual struggle resumed. I intervened in a firm tone of voice: "What you need to know is that God will remain victorious. And with God and within HIM you too will be victorious. All you need to do is to surrender to God." She beamed. "Thank you."

As spiritual caregivers we seek to bring understanding to the two major questions of spiritual struggle (ego versus God/ the divine; God/the absolute/good versus evil). If we understand patients' experiences on their behalf, the scenario often dissolves in the patient without them needing to understand themselves. In one case that means resistance, in another surrender. It is sufficient for them to gain confidence in the spiritual caregiver. Trust and understanding reduce their stress.

Yet why do so many people experience spiritual struggle, darkness and torment at the end of their lives? Who must undergo such experience? This question is common among palliative and spiritual caregivers, physicians and society at large. Regrettably, it is widely believed that the end-of-life struggle is a sign of denial, fanaticism, one's own shadow, or other detrimental aspects of a person's life and attitude. I refute this view based on witnessing many transitional experiences of patients who have accepted their situation with great integrity. Observation tells me that this phenomenon can also have to do with the peripheral or liminal sphere of the sacred, of God or the divine. Spiritual struggle and dark experiences are also often demanded of and granted to those capable of gaining insights into the dark and magnificent dimensions of the mystery.

Nils, a patient in his mid-thirties and the father of a daughter, became repeatedly restless in the final weeks of his life. He tossed and turned in his bed. Then he seemed to force his way through an inner obstacle. His nurse and I offered him our hands as resistance and encouraged him to continue his efforts. All of a sudden he became still. His daughter had come to visit. Did she make him happy? He remained calm. Could he see anything in particular? No reaction. A while later, he was fully present in the here and now, and I asked him about his experience: He had seen a fireball, similar to the sun, but it had been a ball. It was evident, he said, that this ball would take care of Janine (his daughter). He shook his head. What could it have been? My interpretation of God as the epitome of energy made sense to Nils. And yet he said: "But the ball was repeatedly surrounded by complete darkness. Did this have to do with the otherworld?" He shrugged his shoulders and looked at the nurse and me. My interpretation of "spiritual struggle" caught his attention. "Yes, but why does this happen precisely to me of all people? After all I accept my death." I explained the phenomenon of peace before death and that this was often preceded by struggle, which even those with a strong personality experienced. He had evidently been granted insight into the mystery of the divine (the fireball, energy). Nils relaxed and grew calm. He drifted away into a state of absence. He murmured something. Two days later he died peacefully, in the presence of his daughter.

Chapter 6

Experiences of God and the Divine

The contents of spiritual experiences lead us to the heart of mysticism and religious dialogue. The mystics described the mystery of God in different ways (Lutz 2011). Mechthild von Magdeburg (1207–1282), for instance, spoke of the "flowing light of the Godhead" (Keller 2011a: 71). Meister Eckhart (c.1260–1328) dispensed with descriptive categories and instead maintained that experience occurs without reason and in no particular manner (Keller 2011b: 76). Jakob Böhme (1575–1624) referred to the *Ungrund* (abyss) and meant the "unmanifested God beyond all differentiations," "quite simply the indeterminate and indifferent," "the eternal One," and "eternal Nothingness" (Rusterholz 2011: 104; Rohr 2009).

The Experience of Unity and Being

Dare to leap into the abyss,
blinded, amazed, and freeing yourself.
Free yourself from all earthly shackles,

lose yourself and tumble into nothingness.
Whoever falls boundlessly, has become boundless
And the center of all being,
Of the turning wheel,
which makes us motionless
and one![1]

Mystics throughout history have sought to describe states of unity and being. Ruysbeek's description refers to Logia 74 and 75 of the Gospel of Thomas, in which mystical union is a prerequisite for entering the wedding chamber of God."[2] Modern patients describe such states similarly: *"At one with the cosmos," "Whole and complete, as if no division had ever existed," "Being instead of doing," "Time seemed to have become full and complete," "The present," "Vitality and yet calm," "All and nothing."* The experience of unity is all-encompassing: nothing goes astray, nothing is lost. This state of being is eternal and full (in the sense of the "fullness" attained). Neither a beginning nor an end of being is evident, nor any opposite positions and ambivalence. There is just a state of being beyond space, time, causality and ambivalence that eludes our understanding. Even the tension between good and evil seems to be absorbed into this state of being and thus surmounted. The feeling associated with such experience is often described as a state, a being or a peculiar freedom: We are no longer burdened by concrete worries. Also our ego-centred identity and self-determination, our ego-centred claims to power become superfluous amid our experience of all-embracing connectedness and participation. The experience of being is described as intense, sensuous, and at the same time beyond sense, as a pure presence (Rohr 2009)

---

1   Erik von Ruysbeek, mystic and poet (not to be confused with the medieval mystic Jan van Ruusbroec), referring to Logia 74–5 of the Gospel of Thomas, Ruysbeek and Messing (transl. 1990/1999: 136).

2   "(74) He said: Master, there are many around the drinking barrel, but there is nobody in the well. (75) Jesus said: There are many standing by the door, but only those who are alone will enter the bridal suite" [single: those who "achieve unity and singleness"]; see Davies (transl. 2002: 96–7).

that encompasses the past and the future, a state in which we have overcome the limitations of our bodiliness (Grof 1991; Jäger 2002). Here are some examples:

> *A few days before his death, a young patient described the following experience that he had repeatedly when listening to Koto music: "It was simply wonderful. Grief no longer mattered. Time no longer existed: Everything was like a great Being, and I was so united that I no longer felt I would have to die all alone. My little son was also with me—and yet he was not. Even my afflictions have lessened."*

> *A motorcyclist who had suffered a terrible accident told me: "In those seconds of the accident, time became eternal. I could see the past, present, and future all side by side. But not only time was simultaneous but so was space: I saw my motorbike, the truck and a great light all at the same time. The light, which was next to me but also inside me, surrounded me entirely in the intensive care unit. The light had always been there, and I was there—and yet I was not really there. It was a great, indeed an enormous being."*

> *The life of another terminally ill patient, Simon, had been marked by drug abuse and prison. He sometimes experienced an inner freedom, even in prison, "like a monk in his cell." Then again the shadows of his misdemeanors had hung over him like a curse. Now he was experiencing music-assisted relaxation: "'Pure, unadulterated, magnificent light. I feel at home in this light, at one, as if in another world." He knew this feeling from his former monastic freedom and some exceptional drug-induced trips. One took upon oneself nine false trips and shocking torment to experience this particular light just once. He asked, "Please could you play this light again for me!" "No!" I replied, "I don't want to support your trips." Instead I spoke about spiritual experience and about God as the backdrop to all human longing. Simon was familiar with*

the notion of God as light. The light and this interpretation comforted him, also for the coming time of darkness.

A young female patient told me: "My body felt vast, full, and empty all at the same time. Somewhere my body ceased and merged into the surrounding space. I felt warm, comfortable, as if another substance were flowing through me. The pain was gone."

After music-assisted relaxation accompanied by tubular bells and an arched harp, a female patient said: "It felt as if my upper body had gone. My legs, which always hurt, were still there, but differently. Nothing hurt. Everything, within my body and without, felt incredibly free, out of touch and yet present, in touch."

A tetraplegic male patient told me: "Now I am, whereas before I was always waiting." For days he was simply happy.

Critically ill patients repeatedly report such experiences, after which they live radically in the "here and now." As one patient told me: *"Only the present matters now. Every single moment is life, is almost spiritual."* Experiences of unity often induce the deepest possible relaxation and pain relief. Sometimes, such experiences are intuited as the most extreme earthly state:

A technician about 60 years old, suffering from cancer and who was not expected to die soon, had a dream: "It was as if I were turning more and more into a skeleton." He made large circular movements to illustrate that this skeleton, and thus he, was dissolving into "a wonderful cosmic unity." Sharing his dream with me moved him deeply and he added: "But it was more than heaven or angels." He was discharged from hospital a while later and died suddenly at home.

Roundness (circular movements) is a metaphor of the divine, of the Whole, in which everything is contained and where nothing is superfluous. Where everything forms a Whole, the

Whole is also the One. Then, no "secondness," whether beside or beyond the One, is conceivable. The images of such complete being transcend the human imagination and logical reasoning. Wholeness and Being are concepts of God/the divine, albeit less in terms of power than in a state of being (on the concept of God/Godhead, see the Introduction, footnote 2).

Whereas the divine is experienced as monistic (as a single whole) in experiences of unity, other experiences of transcendence center on a Thou and are as such dialogic. Whereas the experience of unity primarily describes a condition (being), dialogic experiences convey an event, a process involving cornerstones and interactions, in sum relationship and becoming. In contrast to their noticeable absence from the current debate on spirituality, direct and indirect experiences of a Thou are traditionally far from seldom. They occur in mysticism, for instance, in the form of bridal mysticism (Song of Solomon, Hildegard von Bingen, John of the Cross, Teresa of Avila), or in the absence of God (Mother Teresa, Simone Weil, Jakob Böhme and so on).

The Experience of Otherness

There the angel of the Lord appeared to him in a flame of fire out of a bush; he looked, and the bush was blazing, yet it was not consumed. Then Moses said, "I must turn aside and look at this great sight, and see why the bush is not burned up." When the Lord saw that he had turned aside to see, God called to him out of the bush, "Moses, Moses!" And he said, "Here I am." Then he said, "Come no closer! Remove the sandals from your feet, for the place on which you are standing is holy ground." He said further, "I am the God of your father, the God of Abraham, the God of Isaac, and the God of Jacob." And Moses hid his face, for he was afraid to look at God. (Exodus 3.2–6)

In this particular type of experience something alien confronts us. There is an encounter with an opposing nature. In Exodus, it is the experience of the unknown God without face. The origins of the word "God" emphasize the elusive and relational aspects of that supreme being: "God" is a loanword, whose basic form in Germanic was *gudam*, a neutral participle (Reiterer 2009). Depending on the Indo-Germanic root, the word means "the called upon" (*ghau*, to call, to implore, to invoke), or "the one sacrificed to" and "cast in iron" (*gheu*, to pour). The latter instance is less likely. "The called upon" implies the relational aspect: we invoke God/a supreme being in search of a relationship. God/a supreme being, in turn, seems to be an elusive authority, neither male nor female. In all Germanic languages, "God" became male in the course of time (Reiterer 2009). The inconceivable IT became HE.

Compared to the sensuous experience of a fatherly-motherly God/Godhead, as observed in the next chapter, the experience of Otherness is an older concept in developmental psychology and religious history. Moses's experiences of the burning bush (Exodus 3.1–6) and on Mount Sinai (Exodus 19.1–20) epitomize this experience. To this day, people experience a largely shapeless, powerful counterpart at significant waystages of their lives:

Francine, a critically ill woman of French mother tongue and a deeply religious 60-year-old patient, had to decide whether to have chemotherapy or not. One morning she was still moved by a dream she had had the previous night: "Do you know Moses?" she asked me all of a sudden. Then she told me her dream: "There was a voice. It called my name: 'Francine—I AM WHO I AM.' The voice then said emphatically: 'Viens, viens (Come, come).' It was clear to Francine that she would refuse chemotherapy and that the dream was about dying. And she was certain that death was imminent. Time and again she was enraptured and murmured "Moses." On one occasion, far away from the here and now, she asked me: "Have I already died?" After a few peaceful days, she did.

Experiences of Otherness are extreme relational experiences, involving the encounter with the divine as an authority or as the absolute truth. Such experience is binding, unconditional and leads to the freedom and knowledge that in our innermost conscience we are bound only to God/the divine. Dreamers experience themselves as personally addressed. The experience of Otherness impresses itself deeply on their personality. Such experience "gets under the skin" (and sometimes even causes skin reactions). We are unable to forget the voice heard or experienced in a dream, nor the beckoning eye, nor the finger pointing at us or touching us insistently, particularly if synchronicity is involved. Such experiences confront us with what concerns us directly, sometimes making such encounters unpleasant and overwhelming. In some cases, we try to ignore or devalue, or to reinterpret, such experience. "Well, it was only a dream." On the other hand, it is their depth and inevitability that makes such messages sacred. Such experiences have great potential: answering their call makes us feel guided, strengthened, nurtured. The strength to overcome the unbearable is given to us hour after hour. The sender of such messages remains anonymous and imageless (note the prohibition of images in the Old Testament; see Exodus 20.4). And yet a relationship exists nevertheless. We are recipients. We dream, for instance, about a (professional) vocation, or our dream announces a task, a change of course, a step toward forgiveness, or a moment of deep appreciation:

A young man returned to life from a near-death experience with the inner call "to express even greater love." From that moment, his assignment was identical with his need.

One elderly patient who had a near-death experience, experienced just one feeling: remorse. Coming back, she felt the need to begin a new life.

An elderly patient whose condition was precarious after suffering an accident had the following dream: "I am at a place where strange figures are hanging on the walls." With these figures he associated a pack of cards, tarot reading and fate. "Here life and death are decided. But I don't know by whom. I still have matters to attend to, I am told."

A patient who had caused another woman's death (Joan) in a road accident had suffered from a sleeping disorder ever since. One night she dreamed of a merciful God. "I saw nothing, but heard the following words: take heart, there is space for Joan and you." With some few exceptions, the sleeping disorder stopped after this dream.

Disappointed by one of her children, a mother decided to forget this child, to eradicate it from her life. Her power to love had ceased, she told me, until she had dreamed of her daughter as a young child, who was no more than a pair of eyes, and who had looked at her so imploringly that since the dream she could do nothing but love this child. "This dream has made forgetting impossible!"

In many ways, the experience of an opposing nature amounts to an encounter with the very authority to which we must answer. The common belief in a "Day of Judgment" takes up the idea of an authority over the truth that establishes justice. Spiritual caregiving has led me to a milder, more beautiful interpretation: experiences of a tribunal at the end of life are mostly experiences of *appreciation*. Sometimes, this occurs spontaneously, at other times it happens after spiritual caregivers have managed to express a seemingly crucial appraisal.

He had had a stupid dream, Dirk told me one morning: "There was a chair…and beautiful music." I pricked up my

ears and sat down next to his bed: "Tell me about the music."
He began to, but he did not know why the atmosphere had
been so beautiful. At some point, I asked: What would happen
if he sat on the chair and listened to the music? He fell silent,
tears streaming down his face from behind his closed eyes.
Then he looked at me and said awkwardly: "Here one receives
appreciation." This sounded so abstract that I asked: "How
did that happen? What exactly did you hear?" He replied—
almost ashamed: "I kept hearing these words: 'You have done
so well. So much of what you have done in life, you have done
so well.'" I remained sitting silently next to Dirk, touched
by his account. A few hours later, his family gathered for a
blessing ritual that he had requested. In my prayer, I took up
the words of his dream. Then Dirk ceremoniously blessed his
wife and children—before he drifted away, immersed in a
great act of release, which merged seamlessly into a peaceful
and comatose state. He died a few hours later. Previously, his
doctors had discussed an operation because his life expectancy
was estimated at about two years.

During music-assisted relaxation, another patient saw himself
"just sitting on a chair." Someone—he did not know who—
had pressed a "great letter of appreciation" into his hand. This
patient also died the following night. (In my experience, it is
not uncommon for patients to dream of "a voice that praised
me." To realize, or even just sense, that we are recognized by
God/the divine as the absolute authority is deeply moving.)

This type of experience is, however, not always spontaneously
recognized as an experience of an opposite force. It is a
profound taboo because it is too close, and too overwhelming.
Let me give an example:

Tamara, a young mother and a former catechist, had
abandoned all religious sentiment. She knew me as a music
therapist. On one occasion, she asked me, out of the blue, why
I was religious. Our discussion enabled her to overcome her

resistance all at once and to find her own words. Weeks later,
after her health had deteriorated, she sat before me, her legs,
feet and waist bandaged. She had come to see me about her
lack of spirituality. Her whole body had been trembling for
days. She had goosebumps and a constant itch. Just now, she
recalled a dream: "Well, actually, there was nothing." She
knew that it had been an important dream, but she neither
saw nor heard anything. I asked her what nothingness had
looked like. "Everything was dark, as if there were very many
small drops of dew or sparks of light in the darkness. But they
were so small that it was nothing." I sat up. Perhaps this had
not simply been nothing, but the great Nothingness, which
was an actual Something. Could she imagine what it felt like
for one's skin to be touched by this Nothingness? She shivered
even more. Might her shivering and itching be related to this
experience? I referred to Moses to illustrate that I AM WHO I
AM. Tamara looked at me, stunned, and understood without
understanding. The next day the shaking and itching had gone.

Our experience of such an elusive, inconceivable opposite
makes us feel like a powerless, naked creature faced with an
infinite, unknown stranger. Jacob's struggle at the river Jabbok
(Genesis 32.22–33) brought him face to face with such a
ghostly figure. "…and a man wrestled with him until daybreak"
(Genesis 32.24). According to Maria Kassel (1980: 269–71),
this refers either to a pre-Israelite story of a demonic creature or
to a river god. Ultimately, Jacob experienced neither a demon
nor Nothingness, but God and his blessing. At the hospital
bed, it is not always possible to dissolve a patient's spiritual
struggle. In such cases, patients remain waiting, staring into
the distance, or frozen by their fear of the numinous:

Marc lay on his deathbed, unable to die. For three weeks, he
could barely move nor communicate with the outside world.
I noticed that he was almost constantly awake, his eyes open.
His gaze remained unaltered, lifted upward, and his hand

clasped the grip hanging over his bed. His eyes conveyed an indescribable fear. I did not know whether he could hear me. Only his wife's presence—day and night—seemed to calm him somewhat. Her husband had had a brilliant sense of design and music, she told me, a keen eye for spatial composition and pictures, and an ear for sublime music. The music therapist in me pricked up her ears while Mark made a soft groaning sound, his only sign of life for over 70 minutes. Those words must have been important. What haunted this patient, I wondered.

Back home, I told a visiting professional music-therapist colleague about Marc and agreed to do an empathy exercise. I lay down, adopting Marc's posture: My hand—which soon tired—reaching upward, my gaze staring unchanged at the ceiling. What happened? For a while, I could see nothing at all, a dreadfully cold nothingness. The few visual stimuli in my field of vision had long dissipated. What struck me, however, was the boundary: here was the ego, there the non-ego. Already beginning at the tip of my nose, the non-ego extended into eternity. Now came the impulse: Something alien, and profoundly disturbing, confronted Marc; that is, he could see the incomprehensible without seeing it and it unsettled him, indeed froze him. He was terrified of the numinous.

The next day, I visited Marc. He lay there, his posture unchanged, sweat pouring down his face. I told him about my experience. To his wife's surprise, he replied "Yes" and groaned. I repeated my account and explained that we experience this most fundamental fear as soon as our ego begins to develop (intra-uterine, as a newborn child and as a baby), that is, when the ego and the non-ego become distinct. This separation created the impression of something alien, vibrational, confronting us. "Rrrr," responded Marc. I shivered. How dreadfully concrete must these "vibrations" be for such a musically and visually gifted man, and how threatening the boundary to the non-ego. I said: "Now, as you approach death, you are evidently experiencing the same fear." Another response. The tension lifted for a moment. I became more explicit: "What you are obviously enduring is terrible, but also ingenious. You have taught me so much. If your experience is what it is, you need even more courage to trust yourself to let go and to remain standing amid your fear. Perhaps you could also allow yourself to stop thinking." (Thinking is a way of coping with difficulty.) Marc breathed deeply. His grip loosened briefly, only to tighten once more. Digestive noises. His wife said: "He heard you. I don't understand what you said, but your words have evidently done him good." I tried to relativize Marc's fear of the numinous with a familiar image of God and told him about Elijah at Mount Horeb (1 Kings 19.11–13): God was neither in the fire, nor in the earthquake, nor in the wind, but in a gentle whisper: "The great big thing that you are probably seeing can be tender, a gentle whisper, just as Elijah experienced God at Mount Horeb. Have courage." Marc breathed deeply, and for the first time he relaxed and let go of the grip above his bed.

Two days later, his eyes were closed. He was sleeping, said his wife. Now that he was peaceful, she could also sleep again and bid farewell to her husband. A few days later, Marc died in great peace.

God/Godhead as Father and Mother

The numinous epitomizes what overpowers us and what we experience as "too much." God/the divine must assume manageable dimensions if we are to endure either. This happens, for instance, if we experience the abstract, the atmospherically boundless, as a figure or "face" with human features. Generally, this coping mechanism is part of developing different concepts of God: What is otherwise an overwhelming power becomes non-imposing, a God/Godhead, who grants us space and who protects us in need; he is a reliable ally, a God who approaches us unthreateningly and dwells among his people (Exodus

29.45–46). God's name and essence manifest empathy, as a God who intrinsically understands his people's fate, as a father figure in the analogous sense of the Old Testament. Importantly, JAHWE, the proper name of God in the Hebrew Bible, should be understood less as an ontological concept of existence or as a proper name than as an assertion of God's essence and his work (Kunzler 1998: 159–60).

Is our modern experience similar to Elijah's in the Old Testament? Experiencing a fatherly–motherly deity is not uncommon today. Such experience is already an answer to our fear and common among people with deep-seated fear. The nature of such experiences of parental love conveys emotional security, protection, and loving understanding. Such experience, moreover, is a haven of peace and relativizes excessive strictness. It allows us to be a child once more and provides our inner child with resonance. A sacred text, if heard at the right moment, can induce such experience:

His handshake told me that Walter needed an authoritative distance between himself and others. He was keen to discuss theological, but not emotional issues. Why, however, was this abstract thinker and man of faith reading the same Bible passage time and again in the last weeks of his life: The Lord is my shepherd; I shall not be in want? (Psalm 23.1) He became calm whenever reading these words.

One patient, about whom there seemed to be nothing childlike to begin with, called out for his grandmother as he approached death. I advised his anxious wife to treat and kindly soothe her husband like a grandchild. It worked wonderfully.

One dying woman heard the lullaby "Sleep, baby, sleep" in a dream.

Another dying woman, her face beaming with joy, for hours saw "flowers, meadows—a flower." When she awoke, she said:

"Flowers were my childhood. And just now there was one large tulip. It covered me like a rainbow."

Tanja was aware of her mental decline, brought on by brain metastases, and deeply ashamed of it. When she was lucid, I read the following verse from Isaiah (Isaiah 49.15): "Can a woman forget...the child of her womb? Even these may forget, yet I will not forget you." This verse struck a chord with Tanja, particularly since her mother had been the person closest to her. With astonishing clarity, Tanja continued the train of thought: "A mother isn't ashamed of her child, not even if it is in my state."

Beatrice, an elderly lady, was deeply fearful. It took her weeks just to summon the courage to consult me. Then, one day, we met in the hall: "Now I am ready. But I have to say that I am afraid." She described her restlessness while we walked up and down. What protected her at home? What gave her trust? She was religious to some extent, and often prayed to the Virgin Mary. "Would you like to visit me at my practice tomorrow, listen to music and receive a sign of blessing against your fear?" The following morning, Beatrice, fully dressed, was already waiting for me outside my practice at 7.30a.m. She asked me to make the sign of the cross on her hand and forehead. I did so and spoke these words of prayer: "You are protected in the name of God, the Father, the Son, and the Holy Spirit." "And Mary (the Virgin Mary) is also here," Beatrice added immediately. "Can I pray with you?" Together, we prayed: "I am protected...and Mary is also here." Now she dared to walk out into the day: She bid me farewell, I took off my coat, and turned on my computer.

Later that day, I visited Beatrice in her room. She asked me to make the sign of the cross on her body wherever she felt fear. Then I played some music. She smiled and became drowsy. That evening, the nurses told me that Beatrice was different, calmer: she was repeating her prayer-like sentence to Mary ("and Mary is also here") like a mantra.

A few days later, during a discussion about transferring Beatrice to a nursing home, she was trembling again. What, I wondered, was causing this immense fear? She had grown up during the war: gunshots, scrambling for protection in the air-raid shelter, Russian soldiers everywhere...(I imagined that she had been raped several times). As a child she had been called "Mitzi." "How can you bear all of this," she suddenly asked me, "you must be exhausted." When I denied any exhaustion, she flinched and ended our conversation abruptly saying that she needed to rest. I had to realise that I had lacked empathy. On my next visit, I brought along Psalm 34, which I had written down in large letters ("I sought the Lord, and he heard (answered) me, and delivered me from all my fears" (Psalm 34.4)) and a postcard of the Mother of Grace from Einsiedeln Abbey, with greetings from my father on the back. The gift had an overwhelming effect. Beatrice asked me: "Is your father still alive? Mine was killed in our village when I was a child. Will your father be going to Einsiedeln again?" She closed her eyes, sat before me without trembling, and seemed to have forgotten the passage of time. After ten minutes, she said: "Now I have a new father." She kept the card and the Psalm in a safe place. Not a day passed until her death without Beatrice taking out these possessions, looking at them and affectionately putting them back where they belonged.

What was it that these patients actually experienced? Their experiences emanated from between the lines: a grandmother, a lullaby heard in a dream, a protective flower, an answer to shame, a mantric prayer to the Virgin Mary, the experience of having a (new) father. How such inner connections with the divine occur remains open to discussion. Their effects, however, speak for themselves.

There are, of course, also concrete experiences of a God-as-Mother or God-as-Father. We dream of a great, bearded, benevolent shepherd; of a sweet-tempered queen with long hair; of a soft and gentle lap or home that is more than an earthly house. The dreamers find themselves amid their vision, sheltered, consoled, or caressed. They can fall neither through nor out of such a great lap. On the one hand, such images or associations touch on our experience of socialization and resonate with internalized childhood experiences with the Bible and/or other sacred scriptures. By the way, 30 to 40 years from now, there will be another generation of the dying, one no longer familiar with the Bible, although they may have grown up in Europe or North America.

On the other hand, such profound images not only represent our socialization but are also part of an archetypal treasure and convey the experience of emotional security, primordial trust, or a "deep knowledge" of dying and becoming. Under the sign of the Great Mother, who affectionally embraces all becoming and dying and who even lovingly accepts the fragments of her own destruction, a new intrapsychic and spiritual beginning is always possible. It is as if a great "Yes" stood over and above everything. *Experiences* of God-as-Father and God-as-Mother are deeply life-affirming, in stark contrast to the often distorted images of God/the divine handed down in the course of human history. Such experiences are sensuous and emotional. *"A God who carries and nurtures me, who is pleased when I reach home, who consoles me and is tender, who is gentle and warm."* When we attain such a sense of emotional security and joy, the misfortunes of life and the shortcomings of our barren years are overcome, jealousy is appeased and sadness dissolved.

The next category of experience, which goes one step further, concerns a mysterious presence of the divine even in suffering and powerlessness.

The "God Within": Experiences of Presence and of Christ

Where is God in the greatest suffering? When we feel extremely threatened or past hope, God no longer seems to exist, not even for religious patients. God, or the dimension of transendence, seems lost. Amid prolonged suffering, even persons practiced in meditation often can no longer meditate. Everyday spirituality no longer works. In the hospital context, these are the hours of powerlessness and pain, the fear of surgery, the distress caused by the impending transfer to the intensive care unit or a nursing home, and the expectation that the passage toward death will be awful. The so-called "scanner" induces the fear of confinement before and during computed tomography. Such fears are aggravated by a patient's biographical fears or traumas (violence and physical attacks, war, abandonment). The powerlessness suffered in the past is reactivated by a present helplessness and seems to be out of proportion. Moreover, our present fear is triggered by past feelings of forlornness, shame, and self-depreciation. It has become like an automatic pattern, totally independent of our will. Words of appreciation, which relatives and caregivers often express all too hastily, and pious talk of God, are perceived as empty phrases, as lies and betrayal. As one patient told me: "Don't you mention the Bible. My Bible contains the same words as yours. And you can leave your panaceas at home." Advising patients to simply believe or to let go is often perceived as equally unempathic. And exactly in such moments patients are unable to relax. They feel disconnected from the Whole/the One, from God, and excluded from the good and beneficial part of life. Precisely this heightens their despair. Patients tremble, cling, search, freeze and grow embittered. They need to be understood: What has become total suffering? Our empathy can never be deep enough in such situations. What, however, reaches a patient under such circumstances? Is there still hope? Grace?

In my experience, only *love* reaches patients afflicted with near-total suffering. But what kind of love? First, an empathic love. They need spiritual caregivers and friends, who bear and permit such intensive suffering while remaining silent and in whose presence patients dare to feel their anger at God and their fate. Because solutions cannot be found without considering the question of God/fate, patients often need someone who *asks* them about God/the divine and their emotions, and their feelings of forlornness and betrayal, and who does not shirk these issues. Patients need someone able to endure their suffering amid seeming hopelessness, someone who lends them words for their plight, and most of all someone who is *present*. They need caregivers, and relatives who unmistakably signal that "I really care about you" and who also live this message. This is genuine empathy, of truly being *with* someone (see Benedetti 1992 and Chapter 8).

Second, the love must be transparent, genuine. The suffering need spiritual caregivers who also feel themselves and their limits, up to the point where they too have exhausted their resources. Love, in suffering, does not advance faster than an individual process and situation permits. Caregivers need to engage also with themselves, while keeping open their minds and hearts (for instance, by entering or going into a deep silence or by spending time out in nature, by praying to their God, by questioning themselves in prayer and meditation, by questioning their motivation with a supervisor). In every such "soul-searching," they need to hold on to their hope time and again (see Chapter 3). Often, such an empathic and authentic love must pay the price of surrender. Patients need someone who, while surrendering, loves them anyway and is able to take upon themselves their anger and projections. There is no imperative to love others. The question, instead, is "Who do I love so much that I cannot let that person fall?" I expect that most mothers, fathers, friends, and caregivers know someone they love so much. Only this kind of empathy is able to soften what has hardened in patients during suffering and it is only from such empathy that hope may grow. Such love is never purely human-induced, but also owes its existence to grace. It comes from within us and is mostly born from our own inner resources and spirituality. Spiritual caregivers need profound spiritual nurturing. How would they otherwise have the strength to care for others even in situations of hopelessness? Unlike the aforementioned love, all neurotic volition, however well intended, will fall by the wayside.

When caregivers are as desperate as the suffering, their deep trust manifests itself in their sheer perseverance. Not less, but more groundedness is required, that is, another level on which we are spiritually connected and thus filled with trust and not determined by anxiety. Primordial trust is deeper rooted than all fear, even primordial fear, primordial trust is a spiritual source of being connected (see Renz 1996/2009). Ultimately, the suffering need the coincidence of love, grace, and their own maturation. Such a gift of love has an enormous healing effect: patients at some point feel *being loved and loveable in a fundamental way*, as if they were loved by God/the divine or the Absolute. Such love amounts indeed to a deep experience of God/the divine no matter how patients call this dimension. Patients say: "*I am loved, although I haven't done anything to earn this love*", "*your voice came with me to the examination and consoled me; it was quite simply there, as a gift*"; "*I could feel my wife's hand touching me all the time*"; "*HE/IT(God) was there in the scanner*", "*HE/IT was present in my misery*"; "*there was a light*"; "*a web of lights*"; "*an angel*"; "*Jesus.*" This is what I call the category of "God within," that is, God, a supreme being, a higher power, or a presence amid suffering.

Katrin had long ago once experienced an angel and a light, but she could not retrieve her experience: fear and a deep sense of betrayal by the world and by God had come between that experience and her present predicament. At home, she led a simple life. Her husband, who was retired and thus around her most of the time, was pretty helpless. Despite his helplessness, he achieved something magnificent: every day, he played the cello for his wife, although—in his own words—he was not particularly talented. This was just his way of saying to her, "You mean a lot to me, I love you." Later, Katrin was taken to hospital again and faced a difficult operation. Her fear was palpably total, and sweat poured down her face. I accompanied her as best I could. Then she was admitted.

The next day, Katrin was deeply moved. It had not been bad at all, not even for her soul. She had had a magnificent experience: "I kept hearing cello music, like the music Stefan played to me every day. As time passed, it was as if a luminous figure stood there, more than the angel of long ago, a figure resembling—Jesus."

This category of experience consequentially entails a specific conception of God/the divine: God or a supreme being has become "a savior" or a presence amid hopelessness and suffering, the "God within" us. A synonym for such a concept of God/the divine is love, as mentioned before. This concept of God/the divine, in my eyes, is the epitome of the mystery of Christ, as well as of the mystery of love and deliverance. But it is not confined to Christian religion. Members of other religions can discover similar or other dynamics in their religion. The dynamics presented here seem to have an inherent logic, which can be understood *psychologically*, as a spiritual–therapeutic path that proceeds in three steps:

1. The caregiver, friend, and family member gives himself or herself to another person out of an inner urge; love without lies and betrayal.

2. The caregiver, friend, and family member surrenders, which opens us the person cared for.

3. The experience of grace and transformation (in the one cared for as well as in the caregiver, friend and family member) occurs.

If we want to understand this dynamic, then we must walk this path, step by step. The silent mystery only gradually reveals itself to us and can be experienced only through active involvement. To help us understand this path, I consider it in closer detail below. What exactly do patients—Christians as well as others—tell us about this path, about this category of spiritual experience?

> *Bernhard, who I had been accompanying for a longer period and who had become dear to me, was panic-stricken. He was facing difficult surgery. He was shaking and told me that God helped very little under these circumstances. I was a little bit sad. Could we endure his fear together? He agreed. Then Bernhard was taken to the operating theatre. "Remember, I shall think of you, take these words with you." I was astonished by my insistence. The next day, he said to me, visibly moved: "Your voice came along. But at the same time, it was more than your voice."*

> *Ursina, a nature-loving woman of Protestant faith in her mid-seventies, was saddened by her desolate situation. She did not mind dying, but she feared the increasing powerlessness in her body. She wept for a long time and loved to be caressed. We liked each other. Music and relaxation exercises comforted her: "It was like the music of angels. It came from far away and came very close. My end cannot be bad," she stammered afterwards, obviously consoled. We remained silent. Then she shook her head and could not understand why she was so full of trust. I asked her, "Was there some kind of presence?" (Rohr 2009). She nodded: "Yes, 'IT' was not simply there, it (still) is," she exclaimed. Within the next hours, her symptoms escalated. Her trachea was affected, and Ursula was again afraid of suffocating. A transfer to the regional hospital was planned. I visited her again. She requested music and a blessing. I asked her: "Is there a particular passage in the Bible that you like?" "I love Jesus and imagine him wandering from village*

to village and going up to people." "Could you imagine him coming to you and offering you consolation?" "Why not?" In this atmosphere, I played the monochord and said a blessing: "Ursina, God blesses you. Jesus himself is your companion, as if you were his disciple. He will accompany you to the regional hospital and will place his spiritual hand on your neck, to protect you, and to receive you in death." I played more music. Ursina breathed deeply. The atmosphere was tense. A long silence ensued. Then she cried, but differently than usual. Finally, she said: "That helps. Nothing can happen to me." Two days later, I visited her one last time. "IT is still there. IT helps—Jesus." Three days later, she approached her death (by asphyxiation) peacefully, without any wish for sedation.

Erika, a devout 50-year-old woman, who used to be very physically active, was almost completely paralyzed due to her illness; she had gone blind, was almost completely deaf, but mentally fully present. (Imagine this imposition.) She oscillated between despair and heroic acceptance of her fate. Music and conversations touched her. Occasionally, when I entered her room, her husband lay down next to her, their bodies side by side. I felt embarrassed, until one day Erika told me that she sometimes asked her husband to lie down next to her, because this was the only way she could feel her own body. I was moved by the extent of such affection. Also from me, she wanted my sheer presence: crying together with her, saying a prayer, playing some music, caressing. On several occasions, after music-assisted relaxation, her body felt strangely alive to her (although she was paralyzed!); she felt a physical freedom. After one such musical session she remained silent for a long time. The atmosphere was so tense that I did not dare to speak. In the end, she said softly: "Jesus is here—that's good." This condition persisted for an incomprehensibly long time (days!). Once, when Erika was again desperate, all I could say was: "You are a heroine." She nodded. She seemed moved, only to drift away again. Where to? "Jesus has returned, you know.

Freedom—sometimes one loses sense of time... HE is here."
Three days later, she told me: "My body is—still—fulfilled.
Christ is in me, from tip to toe. I cannot explain how." For
weeks, she lay on her deathbed, radiant. Whoever entered
her room—her nurses, physicians, pastoral caregiver, and
relatives told me—left in a different state of mind. Gradually,
imperceptibly, almost seamlessly, life and death merged.

Such a highly impressive type of experience of transcendence
(God/the divine within), which cannot be equated with any other
category, should not be ignored in the debate on spirituality.
Those pressed hardest rely on us to acknowledge their
experiences and, at times, even to guide them toward an invisible
turning point in their suffering, where grace may happen.
Whereas such experiences of "God/the divine within" were not
particularly frequent among our respondents (33 patients), their
experiences were very similar and associated with profound and
powerful reactions. In our study, for 19 out of 33 patients—
including 5 non-religious patients—the experience remained
effective *for days and weeks.* In 26 patients such experiences
occurred *right at the lowest point of their distress and nadir of
suffering.* What they experienced as *presence* was neither simply
a state (the experience of unity) nor a response (the experience
of an opposite), nor a protection (of a motherly–fatherly kind).
It was more that it was the unbelievable experience that even
God himself or a supreme being shared their plight and was
present amid their horror. *"It is as if HE has exposed himself
to my pain and fear,"* a 60-year-old male patient told me.
These 26 patient narratives can be read as modern miracles,
albeit involving a God invisible to the outside world. In the
other seven patients of this category, finding "God/the divine
within" occurred quietly and silently, or God/the divine was
even permanently present due to previous experiences. These
experiences give us some idea about the unbearable problem of
"God and suffering" (why me? Where is God?) as well as about
a deep mystery of transformation:

An elderly patient of Protestant faith first said: "All my life I have thought Good Friday might just as well be taken off the calendar. Now, I can bear only this God, who cannot help me even if he wanted to." And after a few minutes: "God is dead." Later on, after he had experienced the incredible and dedicated love of his daughter, he described a movement of resurrection: "HE (God) is alive inside me; HE is rising within me."

One young female patient, who had religious faith, was first totally desperate. Then, she had the following dream: "I was in a market teeming with temptations. I felt dizzy and moved away from the hustle. Then I heard the sound of flutes and an increasingly distinct Easter Hallelujah. I joined in the singing, and my voice sounded like in a grand opera. I said: 'YOU are singing in me, from within me out into the world. I am literally being pulled into life, where I belong.'" The dream had resonated in the patient for three days. It was as if I was sitting opposite another (new) woman.

A young Muslim who was familiar with Sufism was ashamed because he felt he had lost his honor amid his illness. Shortly afterwards, he was full of divine energy: "Strangely enough, I am experiencing a light. I feel more alive than ever, although I am terminally ill. The light streams through me."

A non-religious man about 60 years old was embittered because of his illness, symptoms and pain. "If there were a God, he would laugh about me." However, the specific empathy of one caregiver (a nurse, who was not too gentle, but reliable and fully committed) and the loyality of his wife touched him. One night he remembered his own near-death experience years ago, and the experience was acutely present: "There was one great light, I don't believe in God, but this was nevertheless God. And now the light is in me. Strange." He was touched and gentle for days. Less pain, less anxiety.

All these patients felt at loss with a concept of God or a supreme being formulated solely in terms of judgment and power. They could bear only a God/supreme being who knows what such a predicament feels like (note the motif of the wounded healer in this respect). According to Dietrich Bonhoeffer (1906–1945), the German Lutheran pastor, theologian, and anti-Nazi dissident, God allows himself "to be driven out of the world onto the cross; God is powerless and weak in the world and he is with us and helps in precisely this particular way" (cited from Jüngel 1992: 79). Bonhoeffer refers to Matthew 8.17 to illustrate that Christ helps us not through his omnipotence, but through "his weakness, his suffering." Powerlessness, for Bonhoeffer, does not contradict the power of God. It is rather a possibility for God to become present through love (Jüngel 1992: 279–80). Is this sheer consolation amid suffering? Our answer to this question is in fact a matter of personal faith and even more. It does not only depend on attitudes, but also on the experience of transcendence amid suffering. From an experience-based perspective, it is precisely the terminally ill who teach us about this category of "God/the divine within." This does not mean, however, that I consider the mystery of Christ to be exhausted, not even for religious patients (see further Renz 2008a, 2013a; Rahner 1960, 1969, 1984; Schwager 1996).

In discussions about spirituality, mysticism and psychology, I have often been confronted with the following objection: are such experiences not a blurring of boundaries, a human overidentification with God/the divine? This question is crucial whenever spirituality is at issue. It is crucial to perceive God/the divine as fundamentally and forever different from ourselves. Theologically, this means recognizing and accepting difference. The individual should not confuse himself or herself with God/the divine, not even secretly, and not even if the term used is "a higher power" or a mystical union. It is never the ego that becomes God or omnipotent and that considers itself to be larger than itself; rather the mystery or the divine has entered the human, "singing out into the world from within me," as one of the aforementioned patients asserted.

> *An educated man reported the following experience: "It was like a great approval. It wasn't anything imagined…and yet precisely as if God were identical with me, although I was only a part."*

In this experience, we remain radically dependent, presented with a gift. Not we decide over God/the divine, but our identity "comes into being" through him. In practice and in spiritual care: a reverent tone of voice helps to distinguish the nuances.

> *Teresa had been confined to her bed for years. The first time we met, I had 25 minutes to introduce myself between the rounds and her examination. She was desperate, a woman suffering from cancer-induced progressive paralysis (of her legs, arms and torso), which could continue for years. I entered her room and found Teresa unable to move, weeping and trapped in her suffering. If I could, I would have turned on my heels and run away. Then, Teresa whispered: "I am Teresa and who are you?" Her words reminded me of where I was and made me even more desperate because I realized that she was mentally fully present. I introduced myself. Teresa wept and complained of a headache. "May I?" I asked her and touched her head. "I am here. What you are enduring is too much to ask of anyone." "Yes—God…," this deeply religious woman whispered. "What you are enduring is an amazing achievement. You are a saint. I read a lot about saints as a child, but now I have met one." "Hm." Whispering, she asked me why her perseverance was an amazing achievement. After all she was doing nothing and had to cry a lot. We began talking about the meaning and pointlessness of her life. She agreed with some of my thoughts, for instance, "God is just as powerless in the face of your suffering as you are; in fact, he even depends on your inner path, indeed, your courage." When I mentioned that "He delights in you," she beamed and smiled. She sighed again. Then I asked her*

what went through her mind all day long. She said loudly and clearly: "It is as if I had to begin each and every day by taking a decision." I was astonished. "Why decision?" "It is about acceptance." Then, she repeated my words like a mantra: "God delights in me, Teresa." For a brief moment, her mood lifted and she laughed. Then, she revealed her secret: "If one lives as I do, everything is religion. Praying is my day. That is the 'decision' I take to start my day. I cannot run away from God. But no one has told me that he is pleased with me. That makes me happy, from tip to toe, even though I have lost my feeling in my toes." She asked me if she could also pray for me and if I could tell her about myself. At the end of our conversation, I thanked her for all the wonderful things that she had taught me. She continued: "If I don't know what to pray for, I pray my name: 'Teresa.'—That saves me from sinking, you know." The transcendent character of this experience manifested itself in the transformation of her emotional state: she was full of thankfulness, joy and peace for days.

Such experiences are comparable with isolated reports that reach us from the world's poorest: the spiritual solidarity among disenfranchised slum dwellers; the incomprehensible closeness to God/the divine of some people in detention or in concentration camps, and of some torture victims amid their torment. This phenomenon has to be understood as more than mere dissociation. It is not only a psychological, but also a spiritual reality. And here lies the greatness of important Jewish and Christian assertions about God: he is a God of empathy, a (sympathetic) God, who hears the lament of the suffering.[3] *Shekinah*, the term in Rabbinic Judaism for "the indwelling or settling of the Divine Presence of God," also describes the experience of God/the divine "in the midst" and of the Spirit (see the following category). God dwells among his people and

---

3   I am not an expert on the concept of God amid suffering in other religions, but invite an open interreligious discussion.

nevertheless remains entirely sacred, concealed from the view of mortals: he is both the presence and transcendence of God. In Christianity, whose "logos is a person" and whose "savior came down from heaven and was crucified," God becomes "identical" with human creaturely existence and with those profoundly lost. It is precisely in this way that God/the divine restores dignity to the poorest, to some so that they can live, to others so that they can die. I am deeply convinced that each and every religion can find its own tenet of faith corresponding to this category of experience. This could be the basis for renewed dialogue between different faiths.

Experiences of the Spirit

Even today, people experience transcendence as a "Spirit" or holy spirit. *All* spiritual experiences are somehow born of the Spirit. The divine epitomizes energy and becoming. God happens (Jüngel 1992). In our study, this category— experiences of Spirit—was the last one to emerge. Numerous patient experiences could not be assigned to, or went beyond any of the aforementioned, already existing categories. For instance, "a flash of lightning, after which everything assumed a new energy," "a deep movement through the body like trust arising," "an upward movement," a vision, a foreboding, an eschatological feast (including the image of the fireball discussed earlier on). Characteristic of this type of spiritual experience, be it energetic or gentle, is an insistence or urging, a dynamics, a becoming, transformation, movement, a flowing through, a luring out, a being-drawn-to. Experiences of the Spirit are common: 49 patients had such an experience, sometimes among other types of experience. Some encountered the Spirit present in creation and nature, the breath of life, *ruach* (female), just as in the Hebrew Bible:

Zita, an about 30-year-old woman long suffering from cancer, was in constant pain. She experienced highly nuanced and intense impressions of nature, barely like any other patient: sailing, the beauty of flowers, the chirping of birds. These impressions made her feel as if she were in heaven. It was nature and yet so much more, she intimated. She was devout— but in a different way. Later, during music-assisted relaxation, Zita experienced herself as enlivened by the sound of the ocean drum and the lyre. This music penetrated every pore: "I felt carried aloft. There was a great shining light, as if I had been called back into life." She asked me anxiously: "Was it the sun that shone into the room so strongly? Did that cause this bright light?" It was actually raining outside, leaving Zita even more impressed. She added: "Then it was the inner sun. It shone so very brightly." Her experience was an "experience of the world," but with a sense of being called into life, and perhaps even more than that. Was this a foreboding? She soon felt better and was able to return home to live with her illness in a new way.

Jennifer, a middle-aged, apathetic, depressed black African woman, had not uttered a word for days. When I visited her roommate, who at some point asked for Holy Communion, I heard a voice from the neighboring bed call out "Communion, Communion." I placed my chair between the two beds and included Jennifer in my prayer, not knowing whether she could understand me. Both women received Holy Communion. Jennifer merely looked at me. The atmosphere was tense. Then I sang "Amen," a Gospel melody. Jennifer began singing in full voice, with an English accent. The two women got out of their beds, embraced, and wept with joy. The depression was gone—for weeks.

The experience that "Spirit," hope and peace are stronger than the demonic, despair and struggle is also an expression of a greater spiritual force. Not only is this force the effectuating energy "behind" the experience, but it also epitomizes intensity in the here and now, and in a "taking-place." Richard Rohr speaks of the "naked now" (2009). Amid the anxiety and despair, a hidden, purposeful ministry of the (Holy) Spirit—which can be recognized only retrospectively—can assert itself: a Spirit that does not rest until those miracles of transformation *occur* that take place nowhere as frequently as at the limits of life and as we approach death. Of those patients who—besides beautiful experiences—endured darkness and struggle (56), 40 experienced tangible resolution in the end. Whereas resolution was not immediately evident in the remaining 16 cases, it could not be ruled out either. Who knows what comes to pass in the final minutes of life? Where do time and space begin, and where do they end? What does consciousness mean, and where are its limits? Is there endless consciousness (van Lommel 2010)? Nothing is more hidden from view than the inner events occuring *in* dying. Here are some examples of resolution brought about by the Spirit:

> *Antonia, a mother of five and traumatized by violence, lay restlessly on her deathbed. Was she afraid? Only I knew about her traumatic past and could understand her restlessness. My spiritual service consisted of being with her inwardly: saying nothing and yet sharing all I knew about her. Without divulging any details, because her children were standing around the bed with me, I told her: "I am here and both of us are in large safe hands." She seemed to hear me. She first remained restless, but suddenly her body jolted and she became visibly totally calm. The atmosphere had changed. "She is dying now," one of her daughters said. After a few minutes of utter calm, which deeply moved those present, Antonia exhaled. Was this an experience of transcendence or not?*

Karin, an 80-year-old former jazz singer, requested music therapy. Her health permitting, she came to my practice and—dancing, singing, and playing the xylophone—she let her frail body be entranced by blues rhythms: jam sessions in a dressing gown. For Karin, the session was sheer bliss, for me, despite my enthusiasm for jazz, it was also embarrassing, because I knew that waiting outside was death itself. Although her condition worsened, Karin was still unable to die. I visited her at her deathbed. "No, I dislike relaxing music; I want to live…and listen to groovy music." Did she know about her approaching death? She waved my remark aside and dozed off as she made this gesture. She was so exhausted that, however much she tried, she was overwhelmed. On my next visit, I brought her a red flower, but declined her request for jazz music. Karin gave me an angry glance, but because she was so exhausted, her eyes shut again no sooner had they opened. The next time she was so tired that she only said: "We'll play later, won't we, Mrs. Renz?" She grew more and more confused, and talked in metaphors (see Renz 2015, Chapter 5). Was this a means of protecting herself, that she could find the transition across to the other side in a symbolic way instead of confronting herself in a conscious manner? Later, I encountered her in the midst of a vision. She stammered: "I am being picked up. My parents are here. But I need to put on my festive dress. It's going to be a grand feast." "Do you think that we will play music together there?" "Yes, plenty of beautiful music, but differently." The atmosphere no longer embarrassed me. On the contrary, it felt magnificent. Minutes later, once again lucid, Karin resisted her dying. Her resistance was followed by a bout of pain. She was not yet ready for the "grand feast," I thought to myself. She had still not "had" enough life: "To Have or to Be" (Fromm 1976), that is the question. Nevertheless, in her quest for intensity she had attained a very personal sense of fulfillment: a grand feast. A few days later, she died peacefully.

Her unconscious vision of the grand feast had made it easier for me to put up with this clownish elderly lady.[4] Looking back, I realized that in this unredeemed woman a profound urge toward intensity and fulfillment had confronted me. What had never happened during Karin's life and performances still urged itself toward expression on her deathbed. The eschatological feast, to which everyone is invited, is the prototypical image of a "taking-place," a culminating experience at the end of life. Other patients also envision a feast, for instance, as an experience of love or as a wonderful experience of community. Behind such visions stands an urging Spirit. The work of the Spirit is not accidental, nor undirected, but intentional (Sudbrack 1999: 261). It is as if something were striving toward a goal as yet unreached. This phenomenon, which is difficult to explain, occurs at times at deathbeds. We do not die until "it" happens: until the disunited have made peace with each other, until a solution has been found for a difficult child, until the mental legacy has been made for the children left behind, until forgiveness or esteem have been voiced. Precisely this makes families companions in distress, sharing a common destiny, at least for some hours and weeks. Everyone knows that the strength for reconciliation emanates from the person dying.

A man lying lifeless on his deathbed responded "Rrr" to a remark of mine that I had made to his relatives. It was clear to those gathered that he had spoken. Whatever is said is important and so I said to the patient: "Your children and wife are here. We have talked about forming a covenant in this difficult time." This comment animated the man. Each child tried to say something to him, and he even responded by shaking their hand or stroking them (!).

---

4   In her discussion of the archetype of the wise woman, Riedel also considers the clownish old woman and the undignified elderly female (1989: 11, 169–175).

"I can no longer pretend that I did not experience this," a mother told me about the transformation she had noticed in her daughter's dying process. "Since this experience, our life is new, better, although she has died."

Forebodings and deathbed visions, it seems, are also brought about by the Spirit:

Gerd asked not to be served any more food and said that he would die in five days. No one believed him. Everyone assumed that he would live for another few weeks or even months. He died on the fifth day.

Charles, a 75-year-old man, wanted to be admitted to hospital as an inpatient against his family's wishes. There were no medical grounds for his request: his tumor was still small. One of Charles's relatives, with whom he had fallen out long ago, worked as a doctor at the hospital. Charles was aware of this. However, did he know why he wanted to be admitted to hospital? Or was his dying unconsciously intentional—as a work of the Spirit? He made inquiries where his relative worked in the hospital. He approached the "accidental" encounter with somnabulistic single-mindedness. The meeting had been a gift from heaven, he said afterwards. After the second encounter, he said to the nurse that he was going to bed now, in order to die. Could she stay with him? She did—and he died.

Ahmed, a devout Muslim in his twenties, lay unresponsive on his bed most of the time. His wife knew that he would die, as he had told her. He would not die at home, and it would be a Friday. Nor would she be present, but she need not worry. Her husband had seen (in a vision) how things would happen and that all would be well. Ahmed died—unexpectedly for those unfamiliar with his circumstances—at the foreseen time, in that half an hour during which his wife had left his room to run some errands.

The events reported in the above examples could not have come from a knowledge and aspiration located in the ego (Lommel 2010), but only from a place beyond it. Whereas we can hardly explain such phenomena, they nevertheless happen from time to time, particularly to persons open to a sphere beyond themselves and to the workings of a greater Spirit. In our study, five patients, including three very young people, had an actual vision.

Daniela, a 23-year-old woman, who was not particularly pious, was on the verge of dying. The first time I saw her, her mother was present. The silence filling the room felt heavy. The three of us were sad and yet calm, because Daniela was unbelievably relaxed. She liked the silence. Something incredibly mature approached me in this woman, who accepted her dying while also enjoying her last few meals (including a hamburger). She was not afraid, she said, and added that she was allowed to die. We looked at her with astonishment. Soon, Daniela was absent most of the time, oscillating between a comatose and a waking state. The atmosphere was intense. Finally, she pointed at the wall opposite her bed, where an art postcard was hanging, and explained: "Over there…I sometimes see Stefanie (her sister) and then a light shines through the card. It is coming from far away. It is beautiful. Then I only see the card." We remained silent. Suddenly, she stammered aloud: "Light—the light," and then, more softly, gazing at the card, "I see how the world will continue—so beautiful." She gesticulated and drifted away into a comatose state taking the secret of her vision with her. Daniela lived another four days, mostly comatose, and then died.

The Spirit "draws us far beyond ourselves" (Rotzetter 2000: 21). Visions such as Daniela's have led me to wonder about where exactly we are going and about our path toward that final goal. Visions refer implicitly to an evolutive concept of both humankind and God, who is himself "in a state of becoming"[5] (see also Teilhard de Chardin 1955/1959), that is, to the divine, which is evolving. Keller (2008: 23) writes: "*God*, at once eternal and becoming, is a living process of interaction." It is a fundamental statement: The (Holy) Spirit strives toward a goal.

---

5   See the avowal of Rahner, that God/the absolute not only exists but also becomes: According to Klinger (1994), incarnation has a comprehensive meaning. It turns the transcendence that is God/the incomprehensible into an earthly fact. "It is a reciprocal event. God becomes more and more God, and the human being becomes more and more human" (40). Furthermore, "God not only *is*, but He can also *become*" (41; original italics—transl.). Moreover, citing Rahner, Klinger observes: "He who is *per se* unchangeable can begin to change in light of the other" (Rahner 1960: 147—transl.).

Chapter 7

Being or
Relationship?

Is God, is the divine, something or nothing? Is HE/IT
substance or energy? Does coincidence or order prevail in the
end? These questions do not bother the dying. Given their
spontaneous experiences of transcendence, there is no question
of true or false. Patients just have their experiences. Moreover,
patients often have their very own experience of the mystery
of God, of a supreme being and higher power, of the divine
or sacred as an answer to their innermost questions about
their particular situation and distress. This, as such, is *their*
truth. The categorization suggested in Chapters 5 and 6 (five
experiences of God/the divine and two liminal experiences of
the divine) emerged from a phenomenological approach to
patient testimonies (see Renz 2011/2014a, 2000/2008b).

The question of truth is only important in discussions about
religion and spirituality, and for those seeking a promising
meditation or prayer practice. The question presents itself
differently in the various schools of spirituality and religion.
The individual may waver between an Eastern, Sufi, or
Western spiritual tradition. Does it matter which tradition we
choose? Does it matter what is practiced and aspired to in *this*
tradition or *that*? These enquiries raise a systematic question

about conceptions of God/the divine and about an "ultimate goal." Understanding different ways of thinking and faith, as well as their inherent consequences, will improve our spiritual end-of-life care.

The Factor of Formative Influences

Religions are an existential answer—but to what exactly? Conceptions of God/the divine are conceptions of humankind that have grown from individual and cultural–collective developments, from conscious knowledge, from semi-conscious intuitions and from even more unconscious formative influences of a cultural history that stretches back to the earliest stages of human development. Religions hand down their specific conceptions of being, salvation, emptiness and God, the beginning and end of life, and the meaningfulness of humankind and evolution. Can religions and spiritual notions be compared with one another and merged into a new conception? Do such attempts, despite the best intentions, not often risk diluting the religions or falling victim to hubris? Self-made spirituality programs and harmonization attempts divert attention away from the fact that concepts of salvation and cultural answers to the final questions, which each religion has brought forth over a millennia-long development, cannot be exchanged at random. Buddhism, for instance, is a response to a completely different human condition and entirely other formative influences than the three Abrahamic religions. Importantly, although these religions—Judaism, Christianity, Islam—are essentially rooted in the same tradition, they were formed in different historical periods and contexts. They underwent different developments and thus are "in need of redemption" in their own particular ways. Robert Zaehner (1913–1974), professor of Eastern religions and ethics at the University of Oxford, asserted that the principles of Eastern and Western, Indian and Semitic thinking were based on different premises. The sole common denominator of religions is their function in offering redemption (Zaehner 1980: 20).

Religions are culturally specific answers to what consciously and unconsciously determines human beings and the collective in which they are raised: namely, a profound longing, energies and their connotations (for instance, being thrust forward, flowing, or resistance) and above all unconscious fear. Elsewhere, I have spoken of primordial fear (see Renz 2015) or primordial formative influences, and the coping patterns developed in response to such factors, as a background to various forms of suffering (Renz 2008a, 1996/2009). The need for redemption has to be conceived in culturally specific terms—even ethical similarities (Küng, Kuschel and Riklin 2010) fail to reconcile the differences between the various religions.

For these reasons, we must first establish what exactly "a religion" refers to, that is to say, to which specific human and cultural conditions. Only then can we elucidate *how* a particular religion *responds* to these conditions. Only then do we have an idea about the spiritual importance and scope of such answers. What remains concealed in the unconscious darkness of religion must first become more and more conscious and find verbal expression. In all religions, this requires many individuals to strive for, and attain, consciousness. This needs an intellectual, mental and even more an emotional competence: raising consciousness is an emotional challenge, an inner commitment and a questioning of one's feeling and thinking, which involves far more than acquiring knowledge. This also means working on language, that is, finding words for and expressing the pivotal concerns of a religion, its contents of faith and core values.

"Deliverance from our formative influences" (formative influences in addition to and in contrast to guilt) is an axiom common to all religions (Renz 2008a). The claim to find salutary answers is inherent in every religion, and also in atheism. Answers, however, to what exactly? That is the essential question. Religions that reconnect with their roots, their anthropological origins and their formative influences are better able to enter into authentic dialogue.[1] Their pronouncements and rites will also be more and more able to accommodate individual spirituality. Whereas so far I have focused on "formative influences" (including consciousness-raising), let me address a second factor: "the ability to form and to engage in relationships."

Letting Go and Finding: The Relational Factor

Why is an awareness of the different conceptions of God/the divine, and their anthropological–cultural backgrounds, so important? Why is mere tolerance insufficient (you believe this, I believe that) including in end-of-life care? Why is spiritual arbitrariness or randomness (in German I speak of *"Beliebigkeit"*), despite its superficial appeal, no solution? Although openness is important, believing one thing rather than another has inner consequences. No matter how aware we are of the provisional nature of our conception of God/the divine, whether or not we believe in something that transcends us affects our understanding of the self and of the world. Whether or not we believe that this transcendent being turns to face the world and is powerful becomes part not only of our ability to trust but also of our relationship with all being (unlike in, for instance, Pantheism). Whether or not we believe that we can also invoke this force as a "Thou" changes how we deal with ourselves and others amidst distress and suffering. Whether directly or indirectly, these qualities—the conception and experiences of God/the divine—affect our ability to form and to engage in relationships.

Conversely, behind the inability to endure certain conceptions of God/the divine or Nothingness often lie *deeply human, psychological* problems:

---

1   On religious dialogue, see Winter 2013; Renz 2008a: 301–12; Renz 2013b; Rutishauser 2013.

a) The difficulty of accepting the relativity of one's ego and perspective (that is, accepting the fundamental otherness of another religion, bearing to keep open the existential questions, let alone an existence of the numinous). A shaken self-esteem, internalized experiences of being unloved, hurt, and violence, for instance, may explain and compound such difficulties.

b) The difficulty of engaging in obligations and relationships. The difficulty of being loyal.

Both aspects concern our capacity to form and engage in relationships. Not only does this involve more than *actively* approaching others, but it also requires various additional qualities: accepting otherness, permitting encounters with others, allowing oneself to be touched, having a receiving attitude, allowing oneself to be affected by others and a willingness to be part of a larger community and creation— while remaining oneself.

What is called the "ability to form and engage in relationships" on the anthropological level, involves *letting go and finding* on the spiritual level. Several spiritual paths accept the significance of raising and altering consciousness and of letting go and therefore they respond to what has to be left behind, e.g. formative influences, well-established behavioral patterns, enemy images, projections, constraining conceptions of God/the divine. This is important for maturation and for an (unbiased) encounter with God and the divine.

However, where in today's spiritual paths are we taught to practice finding? Where, moreover, are those spiritual paths that, beyond letting go, extend to, yearn for, and indeed even encounter the unknown? And where especially can we learn this orientation to the unfamiliar in the midst of suffering? Where can we learn how to deal with the frisson of touch, our difficulty just to be moved and with deep hurt? Every encounter (with another person, with a personal divine) also includes the inevitable fact of self-correction, which may at first overstretch us and prove hurtful.

While it is the *ego* that lets go (I let go of part of *myself*), "finding" involves accepting otherness and relationship. Finding concerns the "Thou." In essence, it proceeds from the Thou toward finding something. Finding goes hand in hand with encounter, touch, and convulsion. Western culture finds this so difficult because unconsciously it recalls our inate creatureliness (a shaken self-esteem, internalized experiences of being unloved and violence), of the deep wounds suffered in becoming human. Why Western culture is subject to such strong formative influences goes beyond the scope of this book; I would, however, suggest that this has to do with very early human *perception*, with a very early stage in the development of consciousness, with something tragic, but also with a particular sensitivity: called primordial fear (as discussed in Renz 2015, 2008a, 1996/2009). What matters here is that all these wounds concern the *relational dimension* and fundamentally complicate our capacity to form and engage in relationships. Over the course of human development, we have donned protective behavioral patterns from which a dynamics of separation have emerged (Renz 2008a). Psychology speaks of narcissism (Kohut 1979); sociology of the mindset of Western culture being oriented towards having rather than being (Fromm 1976).

What makes finding so difficult? Even more than the act of letting go, the act of finding presupposes that our coping patterns and our protective armor must be forced open, otherwise patients cannot be inwardly reached and touched. It is precisely this, however, that the wounded ego resists: the protective armor and our narcissism, reinterpret our experience of the other. Instead of admitting to being touched or even being ashamed by an encounter, the ego defines it in its own terms: "I decided to meet you," "It was my own idea," and so forth. The other person is turned into and employed as an "object." In Martin Buber's fundamental terminology (1983: 6), projection leads us to perceive an "I–it" in what is actually an "I–Thou" encounter between two independent individuals.

A similar mechanism takes place in every encounter with God/ the divine. We thereby perceive the divine only from the human viewpoint as an object. Vice versa, it is tragic that according to our *conditio humana* only finding, relationship and encounter can/could heal the wounded-cum-narcisstic person from his or her reflexive defensiveness. On balance, risking relationships is our great opportunity and in fact the only thing we can do.

Barbara, an ostentatiously rationally minded woman in her mid-forties, wanted to die. Despite a good prognosis, she had ceased believing in life and its meaningfulness—until one day she was thrown into a spiritual experience: she had witnessed the music-assisted relaxation that I had done with her roommate. She was deeply moved and cried: she did not know what had happened to her. After all, she exclaimed, there had been nothing but sound. And yet she had never before experienced music so materially, so sensuously, just like an earthquake. "Those outer sounds became an inner sound. I no longer felt outside, but within." Unsure whether she ought to find this experience beautiful or terrible, something within her suddenly wanted to live.

Weeks later, she recalled this initial spiritual experience. But her voice was clangorous, her explanations abstract, as if she barely had any space to breathe. Where were her feelings? Weakened by an infection, Barbara was increasingly unable to think. Did she have to die, she asked me. Replying, I asked her whether she could bear not knowing the answer. She stroked me, wept, dried her tears, regained her composure and reprimanded us both: "One doesn't cry." And she asked me to leave the room. The next day, she was waiting for me eagerly; she had a high temperature and was affectionate again. Three days later, she again asked me to leave her room. What lay behind so much ambivalence, I wondered. On one occasion, I mentioned her contradictory relationship behavior. She looked at me briefly and then looked away. The fundamental question of "life or death?" had caught up with her again. Her answer at that stage was "indifference." She loved equinamity in the Buddhist sense. Everything was equally valid, neutral, quite simply free. For instance, at that moment, she no longer knew whether she preferred to live or die. Her voice was shrill, as if she did not feel what she was saying. I said: "Part of me believes you, part of me doesn't." She looked at me astonished. "I believe you that there are wonderful spiritual states, in which one is free, has peace, and that could be described as indifference. I have experienced such states." She interrupted me: "So you do know what I mean. Why or to what extent, then, do you not believe me?" "I don't think that in your case it is about experiencing indifference, but about enduring feelings. If you feel how much you suddenly love life, it is even more painful to bid farewell to it. And you can also sense that we— and that includes myself—care about you. You have expressed various feelings since we first met—closeness, tenderness, rejection, fear—but certainly not indifference." "Feelings are difficult, that's true. I need to think about that," she replied.

On my next visit, despite running a high temperature of 40 degrees, Barbara still wanted to speak about indifference. Her doctor had meanwhile told me that none of the medical therapies prescribed were compatible. Her present infection could not be contained. I told Barbara this and added: "Your body is signalling anything but indifference. It is not at all indifferent to how it is being handled." She reflected, went red in the face, and said: "Correct, I'm seething with rage." I praised her frankness. While enduring anger was difficult, her anger was very understandable. Her face went even redder and was covered in sweat. Two hours later, her fever had gone down. Her doctor became hopeful. Barbara was allowed to live once more. She returned home and rediscovered "a joie de vivre": Nature, music, relationships were all beautiful. Even her body was not that awful, she now believed. Months later, Barbara returned, her voice once again clangorous. Feelings were not an issue. She said she was going to move away to

*live near a meditation center. Meditation was calming. Nine
months later, I heard that Barbara had died.*

Similar experiences with patients give me pause for reflection:
does indifference, the way in which Barbara had understood it,
give us peace? Not only must I leave this question unanswered,
but I can barely comment on the meaning of this ideal for a
person *socialized in Eastern culture*. Quite frankly, Western
culture understands precious little about actual Hinduism and
Buddhism. The problem is our *reckless adaptation* of non-Western
culture to a culture shaped by completely different formative
influences. Whereas meditation may of course lead people in our
civilization to greater calm and centeredness, I am on high alert
when meditative calm is confused with the repression of feelings
or with an acquired rather than a grown sense of freedom. Is
this genuinely a *"redeemed" freedom*? Do people not deceive
themselves when they are looking for aloofness or detachment
in spirituality—that is, a state of mind far removed from earthly
matter, from emotion, and from social relationships? Where is
the boundary between escape (from the world, from the binding
aspect of spirituality) and finding? Where does the need for calm
(*shanti*) conceal a fear of a felt, lived, and demanding life (see the
work of the Indologist Adelheid Mette 2002).

The most profound question is: why do people have such
unacknowledged fear, and what are they afraid of? What makes
relationships so dangerous? Relationships are an admission
of dependence and need! Not only does the longing for
relationship make us realize that we are not self-sufficient and
not only self-determined. It also makes us vulnerable. We risk
disappointment or losing what we love. When we love, we are
perhaps more involved than we wish to be. And that does not
appeal to everyone.

What applies to human relationships is even more true
of our relationship with God/the divine: *"Engaging in a
relationship with God is the greatest risk in life,"* a wise elderly lady

told me, *"because it is a relationship with the incomprehensible. An adventure whose outcome is utterly open."*

So *why*, of all things, is it still worth seeking a relationship with "God himself," that is, the supreme being itself? Generalizations fall short, so let me approach this question through patient testimonies:

> *One 80-year-old patient said: "Perhaps because God is the most profound foundation of all being."*

> *A male patient of about the same age observed: "Because he is the 'truth,' and because I feel honest and sincere when I look him in the face."*

> *A young woman: "Believing in God nowadays is idiotic. I scream at him in despair, and he doesn't answer. But everything is even more terrible without God. It is hollow. If I make an effort to reach him, I feel better. I sleep better, lie better, feel peace. As if there were a gentle answer."*

Uncertainty nevertheless persists. We are unable to establish how we should "benefit" from our relationship with the intangible, nor what or who HE or IT is. All we can do, time and again, is to be startled by our fail-safe, narcissistic shell and by our reinterpretation strategy. Also, we need to realize that scarcely any space remains for unprejudiced spiritual experience. All we can do is to attempt to let go, time and again, and be open to finding. The path leads us backward and forward, through hurt and vulnerability, through our deepest humanity. Those able to affectionately embrace their hurt, accept the protective wall surrounding them and suffer under their own formative influence will experience opening and—if it is allowed to happen—they will find, and experience, grace.

Being and Relationship: The Factor of "Meaningfulness"

From a spiritual perspective, the crucial question is whether spirituality is monistic[2] or dialogic. Do experiences of transcendence concern being or our relationship with God, with the incomprehensible, with the divine as an anonymous "Thou"? Experiences of being denote a mystical participation in a totally distinct state of essence, wholeness and maybe even consciousness. The atmospheric aspect is important. Dialogic experiences, on the other hand, express a final relationship or, more accurately, a state of being related. There is no right versus wrong in this respect. Where in the brain do religious notions (of oneness or of relationship) come into being? What is genuine mystical experience? Nevertheless, and despite sophisticated techniques, faith, spirituality and meditation elude intellectual explanation. Neither medicine nor theology, neither brain research nor neurobiology, neither psychiatry nor the exploration of extrasensory states of consciousness, is able to conclusively explain the emergence, experience or non-experience of such phenomena (Schnabel 2002: 31–2).

Experiences of transcendence provide enough evidence in themselves. Based on my phenomenological studies (Renz 2015) and perspective, I argue that the variety of experiences suggests that *both kinds of experience exist*: the experience of being and of oneness on the one hand, and of God/the divine as a partner in a relationship—and a final relatedness—on the

---

2 Monism derives from *monos*, Greek for "alone, sole, only." Monism is the philosophical view that reality can be explained in terms of a single spiritual or material principle, unlike dualism. In the debate on spirituality, however, another opposition is meant: in contrast to the dialogic, the monistic is understood as what arises from a *single* state or substance. The primary question is: is meditation extended self-experience or does it involve dialogue?

other.[3] Thus, both are in One (or in Nothing), and the One is in both. Above all, every experience of transcendence borders on "mystery."

However, even if we never get to know the final mystery, the underlying self-concepts of these two approaches are very different. Already in the early twentieth century, C. G. Jung observed that whether the human being was related to infinity or not made a crucial difference (1961: 327). Why, however, does the finite not suffice? The human capacity to form and engage in relationships cannot be determined in terms of time and space: where does this begin, where does it end? Love and connectedness are qualities that cannot be compared to material assets. They can never be possessed, but *are* present or not. Even if love, relationship and connectedness are focused on a particular individual, they cannot be limited to this person. Feelings, touchability and atmosphere go beyond all limits. The crucial question is: to be related or not related, connected or disconnected, to risk dependence or not. It is less important whether a human being or God himself, the Godhead itself, is our partner. The challenge is whether or not to become involved. Are human beings able to treat things and to love others, the divine, God? Are we able to become dialogically involved with a "You"? Are we able to function differently than on the level of self-protection, self-determination, having and power? The opposite of connectedness is eventually the need to be in charge, untouchability, hardness and narcissism.[4] It seems to me that a *spirituality of relatedness*—except for some isolated biographies and developments—must first be

---

3   Essentially, the Christian belief in a triune God (i.e., the Holy Trinity), which is in fact difficult to understand, means that relationship is also seen as an aspect of the Godhead itself (between God the Father and God the Son). The Spirit can be understood as the bond "in-between," also between God and the human being (see further Kunzler 1998).

4   Christian theologians like Luther and Augustine speak about human beings curved in on themselves, in other words life lived "inward" wrapped up in one's own affairs rather than "outward" for God and others.

brought into existence, through suffering from excessive ego-centeredness and its civilization. Whether we find our way to such a spirituality of relatedness is—in my opinion—the fateful question for Western culture.

Those Western people *not* shaped significantly by fear and not suffering from acutely severe distress may be able to imagine their life in terms of cyclical becoming and transience: dissolving into nothingness, leaving behind this world without a legacy for the future worth mentioning. Thus, the spiritual experience of oneness can also be understood simply as a dissolution into nothingness. Those, however—like many oncology patients or highly aware and compassionate people—who feel the abysses of life within and around themselves and who endure these chasms to the point of despair, will scream into the dark night: *"But please not in vain!"* *"But please remember the victims of history"* (a fundamental concern shared for example by German twentieth-century theologians like Johann Baptist Metz and Dorothee Sölle, as well as the French philosopher and mystic Simone Weil).

Only a God, only a conception of the divine and the Godhead that recognizes and honors what human lives have become and hears their groaning (Exodus 2.24), who has empathy with them and knows their suffering and helplessness, can be an answer to the individual in his or her suffering and search for identity and meaning. If kept on an impersonal level, such distress can be at best dissolved, but not resolved. The German theologian Roman Siebenrock told me in conversation: "A culture of subjectivity needs a God of relationship." The original notion of a personal God denotes precisely that: the Latin word *personare* means "to sound through, to resonate," just as "it" resonates through me during singing. This means that I am personally addressed by the intangible; it also conveys the message that *"You matter to me. I care about you."* What it does not mean, however, is that we should think of God just as a "person." "Personal" means *relationship*. God, a supreme being, the divine conceived in personal terms is a counter-concept to the accidental, the invalid, the meaningless.

Being and relationship complement one another. Oneness and otherness are *both* part of the divine: they belong together precisely because they are fundamentally different. The experience of being, even if it transcends identity, relationship and otherness does not annihilate them. Or, vice versa, the experience of a divine opposite does not, even from a personal and evolutive–finite perspective, reach beyond and leave behind the experience of oneness. The personal can be completed by the magnificent experience of oneness beyond time, space, and body. Likewise, we can also feel related in the experience of being and oneness. Personally or impersonally, we are part of a whole: held within, healed, based on and connected. Finally, there is *no* answer to the question about the ultimate meaning and the toils of development. The rational discourse about concepts of the divine should not delude us about the key challenge of being open, connected and capable of forming and engaging in relationships. *Every* real spiritual experience affects us personally: it shakes us, relativizes our ego, and initiates relatedness and maturation.

Maturation Sets us Free: Forgiveness, Capacity for Guilt, Finding Home

Spiritual paths are paths of maturation. Time and again, we become open to transformation. On such paths, many people turn away from the church and other religious institutions. But why? There are various reasons: disappointment about institutions and their representatives, a hurt caused by authorities such as parents and teachers, formative influences from one's own culture and the patriarchal *zeitgeist*, an aversion to conceiving God/Godhead as a person or the aforementioned inability to engage in relationships. Hindrances are manifold and are often triggered by internalized primordial fear, especially the fear of the numinous (see Marc in Chapter 6).

The paths of healing are just as manifold. Mostly, they involve long processes of forgiveness, reconciliation and becoming new. "*I have to write letters to the church expressing my disappointment,*" an elderly female patient told me. A middle-aged male patient said that he had "*to literally ask God for forgiveness.*" A young patient said: "*I cautiously made contact with my father again.*" Not only ethical or charitable reasons motivate us, however, but also a need to bring ourselves back to life. Letting go and forgiveness help us to find ourselves.

The question of guilt deserves particular attention: some people dare, at long last, to free themselves from an imposed sense of guilt. Others become, for the first time, aware of their culpability and seek reconciliation. More than 15 years of professional practice have brought me face to face with guilt in many different, indeed contradictory, forms: a convicted criminal lay in one room, in the next room lay a patient tormented by a moral conflict behind which no actual guilt seemed evident. In a third room, a patient thoughtlessly ignored all bad feelings, whereas her roommate wept bitter tears of remorse and simply wished to be forgiven for failing others due to her exhaustion. The biographies of victims stand beside those of offenders and sometimes they fill one and the same book. Some life stories feel like a string of trivial events and yet, with the benefit of hindsight, they amount to a person's silent, understated greatness. The very next person, by contrast, epitomized an overstated uprightness. Thus, the question of guilt polarizes, provokes, and mobilizes. It is hardly surprising, then, that over the past decades a weariness of guilt has frequently drawn people to non-Western spiritual traditions. We have meanwhile largely moved on from questions of guilt. Today, the reason for turning one's back on Western culture seems to shift from the weariness of guilt to avoiding commitment and responsibility—and not least, because there is a lack of convincing Western spirituality and spiritual paths. Wanted: a "spirituality of relatedness" wherein people do not have to be without guilt but are able to feel guilty. This means living with the guilt brought upon ourselves and with our limitations and ultimately allowing ourselves to experience self-reconciliation no matter our baggage. Those capable of feeling guilt know their vulnerabilities. They do not play down their creatureliness and weaknesses. They are prepared to confront their shadow. The capacity for guilt is an expression of a great personality and is associated with a sense of responsibility. Self-reconciliation enables those capable of guilt to place one foot in a more reconciled world and makes them more conciliatory. Their conscience crucially differs from a childlike conscience and from an unremorseful supcrego. Such a conscience is human and under no compulsion to attain perfection. The mature capacity for guilt liberates us from outdated dependence, from a mistaken sense of guilt and from unreflecting guilt impulses (on patterns for coping with guilt, see Renz 1996/2009: 246–8). Persons who are mature in this sense must answer only to an outermost and at the same time innermost source of truth, which affords them charity, freedom, address and judgment (in the sense of reverence and correction). Their final reference of truth is God/the Godhead as the absolute. Truth thus experienced is ultimately greater than guilt. John the Evangelist realized: "…and the truth will make you free" (John 8.32). In our study, the capacity for guilt became important for 40 patients:

> *A dying banker said: "Here I am, I am like this, I cannot do otherwise."*

> *Olivia had been laying on her deathbed for weeks. She had become comatose and unresponsive. I was told that as a young woman she had abandoned her three small children. No one, not even Olivia, knew what had become of these children. Now she lay before me, perhaps suffering, waiting. At some point, I said: "Olivia, I believe that you carry a lot of guilt." The otherwise motionless woman groaned: "Hhh." "I have heard about your three children. We don't know where they are*

either, or what has become of them. But please remember that there is another kind of knowledge. One day your children will understand how you felt at the time and why you left. One day your children will also know that now you are sorry and suffering." "Ahhh." Her eyes were still closed. She breathed deeply and I could hear her rumbling stomach. She died three hours later.

Edith, a former attorney and highly conscientous, was unable to accept her illness. Was she not to blame for her cancer after all? She wept, and I affirmed her crying. She blushed. Other feelings, including anger, also rose to the fore. How could she cope with the question of God, she asked me. I suggested that she express her feelings, her tears, her anger to God himself, to the divine itself. And that she should listen to herself and feel what was happening within. I introduced a body-perception exercise with the words, "Please try to feel what calms you." Edith expressed intense feelings in her body. Her sternum— where her cancer was located—had heard exactly what I had said: "Express feelings," she repeated softly. During my next visit, she exclaimed: "It was like a miracle. God can hear me. I have tried. It sounds strange, but that is what happened and it comforted me." Then she changed the subject: "I keep feeling guilty about my late father, whom I seldom visited in hospital. I was too busy with my husband, who was ill at the time, and the law firm." She cried again. I suggested that she did the same with her dead father: to speak to him within herself, and to reveal her distress to him. She closed her eyes and tried to talk to her father—she spoke, cried, explained, became angry, as if her father were sitting on a chair opposite her bed. She went quiet when I asked her, "What answers are you hearing within?" "Unbelievably, he called me 'Mousey' three times. That was his nickname for me as a child. He isn't at all angry at me." The tormenting sense of guilt had vanished, and instead she was now aware of her own limitations and her father's understanding.

Tanja came to me seeking advice for her terrible gastroenteritis. Without me prompting her, she wondered whether there was something she could not digest. She was having an affair with a married man. Did I object? "It can't be that; everyone does that!" she exclaimed before I could answer. I did not go into the (moral) issue, but instead suggested that she close her eyes and tell her stomach everything she had to say. Her stomach hurt even more, she said. Then I conducted music-assisted relaxation with her. Afterwards, we said goodbye without any further explanations. During our next session, she exclaimed: "I must end the relationship. It isn't right. Even if everyone else does it, it still isn't right." I asked her to close her eyes and to tell her stomach everything. "It's getting calmer. I can see water. It's doing me so much good." She remained silent for a long time. A further relaxation exercise made her body feel different: "I feel a great vastness (she patted her stomach)." The inflammation subsided in the following days. She told me: "I took the right decision. And it helps to listen to my guts."

It goes beyond the scope of this book to explore who has which notion of guilt, or where guilt begins and ends. We live our everyday lives forever uncertain about what is right and what our inner voice asks of us or not. Guilt concerns our own truth and our primordial essence. It is always personal, indeed intimate. No one can teach us about matters of conscience. What does hold true, however, is the prophet Jeremiah's vision of a new covenant:

> But this is the covenant that I will make with the house of Israel after those days, says the Lord: I will put my law within them, and I will write it on their hearts; and I will be their God, and they shall be my people. No longer shall they teach one another, or say to each other, "Know the Lord," for they shall all know me, from the least of them to the greatest, says the Lord; for I will forgive their iniquity, and remember their sin no more. (Jeremiah 31.33–4)

Sometimes, right at the hour of death we are allowed to free ourselves even more deeply from fear and guilt and to find the way back to ourselves, as I once experienced in the case of a dangerous criminal. I have frequently been asked: "How can you accompany a criminal in his dying process? Where do you take the strength from, and the legitimation, to encourage such a person to believe in himself?" Experiences with the dying teach us: *this* very moment offers us the opportunity to let guilt get close to us one last time, to feel it, unnoticed and uncondemned by others.

I find the courage and legitimation to believe in these people especially in their profoundly human reactions at that very moment: the panic-stricken fear of the dying criminal or the deep pain of suddenly realizing what distress one has inflicted on others. Let me turn the question around: am I entitled *not* to believe in a human being, not even in his good dying, that is, to "write off" another person? Citing the fourth-century monk Evagrius Ponticus, the Catholic spiritual writer Anselm Grün (1993) refers to the sacredness of the soul, in which God himself inhabits the human being: "Here he is completely whole, free from all human expectations and plights, free from his own guilt. Here there is no place for guilt…here he is truly redeemed, healed, and whole" (77). Formative influences lie even deeper than guilt. Healing occurs on the deeper level of our formative influences and so do many paths of maturation. They amount to "finding a home" in a spiritual perspective. In most cases, they have a relational aspect:

> *Brigid, a mother of three children, had suffered abuse as a child. This abuse had clouded her concept of God. For years, she had found peace in Hinduism and had lived in an ashram. She was tormented by not having received a sign of life from her son for three years. He had gone missing in Thailand. Recently, not even her affinity with the culture of India consoled her. She returned from her last visit to India feeling betrayed. But she still meditated. I asked her: "Have you ever addressed God*

personally, by name? Have you ever uttered the word YOU in prayer or into the stillness?" "That's impossible: it brings back terrible childhood experiences and the priest's voice." Immediately, Brigid was trembling. For months, our sessions concentrated on giving the trembling Brigid, the adult and the abused child of the past, space and resonance.

Two years later, Brigid consulted me again. She was now fascinated by my suggestion to turn inward to address a YOU. But she did not understand. So I told her a story: "Once upon a time, there lived a man of great proportions. He had a son whom he loved but who was soon committing misdemeanors. Had the father done something fundamentally wrong?" I asked at the end of my story. "Not necessarily," Brigid replied. "Is it right to avoid the father because of his son's dubious behavior?" "No," she replied. I translated the story: The father could be Jesus, the founder of the faith she had grown up with. It was the same with his legacy—of which the Church was a part— as with the misbehaving son in my story. Brigid now began crying, feeling reminded of her own son's tragedy. Just now, a sign of life from her son, who was still in Thailand, had brought her comfort. He had written on her birthday, and was struggling himself. She felt a new hope. Brigid wanted to have a try with the great YOU while meditating. Weeks later, she told me about her profound experiences. She was receiving answers, "including ones that didn't suit me!"

Brigid's case is no exception. Over many years of practice, I have observed that people who experience true rapprochement with their religious upbringing are touched so deeply by this experience because they feel brought back home into their very own realm. While they become religious in a new way, they nevertheless remain themselves. The path through the unfamiliar or foreign may form part of a life story. However, they now return without having to resist for resistance's sake and without the taboo of the trauma consistently excluded from feeling. On the contrary, the other—Hinduism in Brigid's case, and Buddhism, Islam, fundamentalism or atheism in others—now must no longer be a surrogate religion or just an opposite standpoint, but can reveal its very own truth. Interreligious dialogue thus becomes more and more a dialogue between equal but nevertheless very disparate religions (Herzka and Reukauf 1995).

The Path and Remembering a Culture's Specific Potential

Does a culture's "primordial basis" also hold a specific potential? What about a resource-oriented perspective in this respect? Our Western heritage consists of 2,000 years of religious history including Judaism, Hellenism, Christianity, and the Enlightenment. The heritage includes rationalism, a drive towards performance and efficiency, an emancipated approach to basic human rights and a corresponding autonomy, a potential for enhancing awareness and responsibility, and the strong desire for relationship and personal values like self-actualization, identity, dignity, and meaning. In the West, most people are shaped, consciously or unconsciously, by:

a) an evolutive forging ahead and a profound urge toward progress

b) a pronounced subjectivity and a corresponding sense of individuality.

The first aspect concerns our energetic orientation toward the future, the second our understanding of ourselves and of humanity. Both aspects also characterize our "being-in-the-world" and our perception (linear, causal, future-oriented, subjective, ego-related). Correspondingly—but not compensatorily—Western people also need answers to religious and mystical questions.

The first aspect—our evolutive forging ahead—calls for development, awareness, and meaningful goals. God/Godhead, the supreme being is seen as an agent, a creator, as the God of the journey and its detours, even as a perfect being. Conceiving him thus is itself resourceful: over all becoming and life stands a divine "Yes."

The second aspect—our pronounced subjectivity (also known as ego-centeredness)—cannot be equated *a priori* with egocentricity and selfishness, even if it often develops negatively in that direction. Positively, subjectivity reaches fulfillment in personality and in a genuine capacity for relationship. Ultimately, these qualities emerge from our relationship with a "Thou"—specifically, with God/Godhead, the supreme being, the incomprehensible as that "THOU." God/Godhead is the invoked God, the prophesying God and the God of our demand for ethics. HE/IT is a "THOU" to whom the individual answers, but also with whom we struggle and haggle, just as the forefathers of Israel did. Such a conception of God/the divine is resource-oriented: HE/IT takes pleasure in HIS/ITS own person, HIS/ITS existence, and being as HE/IT is. The tribunal, then, means paying tribute!

We experience God/the divine as an opposing force long before we define our personal concept of God/the divine in adulthood. This powerful experience is culturally and perceptually determined. One side-effect of encountering something other than ourselves is a growing sense of isolation and forlornness, and thus an ever-greater fear and the experience of contingency (Drewermann 1985).

Spiritual Experiences of Perfection, Integration, Meaning and Objective

My personal credo is that the final state is not the same as the initial state. Thus, a primordial unified reality needs to be distinguished from the end of the world (Renz 2008a, 1996/2009). Dreamers have a presentiment of the first reality as undivorced, whereas the latter is an entirely different quality of being that approaches us from the goal toward which we strive. Contrariness, identity, relationship and meaning are not simply dissolved in that new state, but instead transcended and placed within a new, otherworldy order (see the evolutive concept of humankind and God in Chapter 6; see also Klinger 1994: 40–1). Occasionally, dreams about the last days of the world recall the images found in biblical parables and the Book of Revelation: namely, the redeemed community and the great assembly of all people and animals, the feast of creation and the music of eternity. The atmosphere in these dreams announces a condition far beyond violence, imperfection and isolation. Eschatological dreams convey our belief in fulfillment at the end of time. The end of the world means more than a paradisiacal–symbiotic oneness, even if this condition resonates with a sense of harmony and emotional security. Eschatological love includes our entire journey, all our endeavors, every distinction, the whole of our personality. Yet whereas characteristics and categories help us to better understand this condition, experience by far surpasses logical reasoning:

An elderly woman, who had felt "out of place" all her life, lay quietly on her bed after a session of music-assisted relaxation. Then she said: "It was wonderful, a great being, a great order, a sea of stars, although I did not really see it. I found myself amidst this order." Moved by her experience, she recognized the connection between "being within an order" and thus "being in order oneself."

Herta, a 50-year-old woman full of life, was moving step by step toward ultimate perfection. The paralysis in her legs, arms and torso was progressive. Time and again, she struggled with her despair to reach a great, life-affirming "Yes." She lay there, released from her suffering, for hours or even days. When I played the monochord, she experienced freedom and light. I had also told her that our conception of God or the divine resembled a loose electrical connection. Filled with light, she experienced that it was gone all of a sudden, only to reappear, to be born from the darkness. Somehow the light continued to shine: "The darkness has gone. Jesus is here. The connection is no longer loose." This condition prevailed until Herta died a few days later.

Hannah was confused: "No, I am not allowed to take Communion. Not everyone has been invited." Did what she saw inwardly resemble an invitation? "Yes, everyone must be allowed to be present, everyone." She cried. I remembered the parable of the wise and foolish virgins who took their lamps and went forth to meet their bridegrooms (Matthew 25.1–13). I also remembered that Communion is a symbol of the community at the end of time (Kunzler 1998: 637). I asked Hannah: "Are there people standing before closed doors?" "Yes," she said, weeping again. I continued our conversation in the language of these images: "Hannah, remaining outside the door and not being able to enter, is a penultimate, next-to-last condition. This makes one cry…but afterwards God once more gathers his sheep, consoles them, and nurtures them as a good shepherd does. Then they will also partake of his feast." Hannah said softly: "Yes—all of them—Communion." I gave her Communion, and she passed away peacefully.

Ros, a catechist in the Protestant Church, engaged me in a theological discussion at our first meeting: "God is disingenuous, otherwise there wouldn't be so much suffering in the world, and I wouldn't have this cancer." She was notoriously restless. Music-assisted relaxation made her astonishingly calm. On my fourth visit, Ros had lost almost all her eyesight. She was sad and longed for relaxation. She felt soothed when I gently touched her hands and stomach. My words that her bed and the floor were carrying her calmed her. She would not fall into nothingness, I assured her. She really seemed to feel carried and let go, deeply. When I mentioned in passing that "Perhaps God is also carrying you," she wept and said softly, "Yes." "Even if you are going to be almost blind, perhaps God is present, invisibly, like a mighty hand that carries us, as we read in Isaiah (49.15–16): "I will not forget you. See, I have inscribed you on the palms of my hands." Ros took a deep breath. Music. Stillness. Then she exclaimed: "It is beyond description, God is really carrying me!" She shook her head, deeply touched: "It is simply incredible. They kept telling us theories about God. And I spoke about God myself. But now I have experienced 'him.'" She remained relaxed for hours. Even months later, she spoke about her experience, still deeply moved.

Ros lay dying. Her family found comforting words, everything was settled, and yet she—meanwhile motionless— still could not die. One afternoon, the atmosphere was particularly tense. What else did she need to be able to die? Appreciation? I suggested a farewell ritual, in which her family and she could express their gratitude. To everyone's surprise, Ros responded to every expression of thanks with "Yes." Digestive noises. Turning toward this dying woman, I explained: "What you are experiencing is the actual meaning of the Last Judgment, whose purpose is appreciation not punishment. This means: 'You have done well. God recognizes and appreciates you.'" "Yesss!" Those gathered in her room shuddered at the forcefulness of the occasion. Her eyes were closed. Although she was no longer able to move, her mind still seemed to be alert. The tension persisted. Was anything else troubling her? "You are probably worried about Peter in South Africa. Please remember that you will soon be close to him in a different way, and that he is well." "Ahhh." The tension eased. I now sang Ros's favorite song, "How Great Thou Art." Her daughters rose from their chairs. Tears, interspersed with "Ah, ah," streamed down Ros's face from behind her closed eyes.

A while later, her daughters asked me to explain the sentence about the Last Judgment and appreciation. While I was speaking, the dying woman commented on my explanation with "Yes." Devastation, a sense of depression. The end seemed near and yet I still sensed distress. I took Ros's hand and said:

"Think back to what we experienced a year ago. A mighty hand is carrying you. No one falls out of that hand. As Isaiah says, 'Can a woman forget her nursing child…yet will I not forget you. See, I have inscribed you on the palms of my hands'" (Isaiah 49.15–16). *Everyone could sense that Ros could hear me. She now began breathing deeply and, summoning all her strength, she leaned her head, although she could no longer move, toward my hand. And thus I held her head. She breathed out deeply—and died.*

Toni, aged 85, dreamed of a city on a mountain. "Unlike now, I was able to walk quite well. There were stairs and low walls, artistic gardens and palaces." Toni's dream reminded me of the Book of Revelation, and so I asked him: "Were there street lights? Was food being served? What were the people doing?" "There were no street lights. It was simply bright. No one was hungry. Everyone had eaten plenty. Lots of people were coming from all directions singing songs." In a subsequent dream, a king was crowned in the city, "a young king was enthroned, and there were many princesses." When we read the Book of Revelation together, Toni could not hold back his astonishment (see Revelation 21: "The holy city…prepared as a bride… Death will be no more; mourning and crying and pain will be no more. And the one who was seated on the throne said…I am the Alpha and the Omega… And the city has no need of sun or moon to shine on it, for the glory of God is its light").

After a long battle against cancer, Fran, a 22-year-old woman, had a deathbed vision. Full of life but bound to a wheelchair, she would contemptuously ask everyone (her mother, boyfriend, siblings, me, etc.): "Do I matter to you? Are you bothered that I will soon die? What will remain of me? How will you remember me?" Dying, she found answers. She did not believe in God, she told me, but she had started praying. She was pleased when I visited her one Sunday: "Have you come to see me?" Indeed, I had, and I had thought about how I would remember her: her cheerfulness, her joy of life despite so much pain. This had given her a finality. Fran, who was drifting away from time to time, opened her eyes, looked at me intensely and closed her eyes again. She stretched her arms toward me and wanted to embrace me. I encouraged her mother, who was also in the room, to find a "final sentence" and to say it to Fran. Fran opened her eyes and drifted away again, her hands folded. The expression on her face was soft. She allowed me to bless her. Fran flinched, and her mother cried. A few hours later, Fran quite unexpectedly uttered the following words: "Not lost, not lost!" I was told that Fran died with her hands folded and her eyes open, looking into the distance.

Chapter 8

Spiritual Care between Psychotherapy and Pastoral Care

Spiritual care has been developed out of palliative care. It addresses patients in hospitals and care homes. Spirituality is often considered to be the fourth dimension in the bio-psycho-social model of care (Pulchalski *et al.* 2009; Sulmasy 2002). Spiritual care embraces aspects such as caregiver–patient encounters, patients' distress, and ritual guidance (Weiher 2012: 1153–71). So far, a practice of spiritual anamnesis has emerged: in many institutions, a semi-structured questionnaire (e.g. Frick, Weber and Borasio 2002) is used to gather information about patients' spiritual attitudes and needs. Interviews are meant to be non-judgmental and patient-centered (Frick 2009b). Spiritual care has sharpened the awareness of the complexity of finding, and having, a spiritual home. Still, reasonable doubts about whether assessment tools are appropriate and feasible in spiritual care remain (Holloway *et al.* 2011: 3). The needs-based approach is just one side of the coin. Spiritual care is also meant to be "spirituality-based," that means, it ought to hope for and be open to grace and let itself be guided by patients' spiritual experiences (experience-based; see Renz *et al.* 2015). Patients' needs and their spiritual experiences are not necessarily the same. Needs often change after a spiritual experience and within processes of maturation, finding meaning (e.g. meaning-centered therapy: Breitbart *et al.* 2010) and dignity (e.g. dignity therapy: Chochinov *et al.* 2005), particularly as patients approach death. Our current study on dying processes (called "dying trajectories") therefore starts from anamnesis and then observes dying processes, including patients' (changing) experiences of transcendence.

Is Spiritual Care Psychotherapy or Pastoral Care?

Who should provide spiritual care? Pastors, psychotherapists, nursing staff, physicians, social workers, or other professional groups? Depending on the authors' outlook, spiritual care is usually assigned to pastors (Weiher 2012) or physicians (Frick 2009a). I phrase the question differently: who should be involved *peripherally* in spiritual care and whose *core competency* suits them to a more central role? This question concerns every caregiver and their educational profile and training. But it also presents them with various important questions: who can endure the pain and suffering of critically ill patients and be open to grace? Who can recognize patient's spiritual experience, who can cope with their spiritual crises and struggles? Which knowledge and skills does this require? And what type of personality? Spiritual caregivers must have two core competencies: the pastoral (Puchalski *et al.* 2009) and the psychotherapeutic. But spiritually sensitive nurses and physicians may also be equipped to provide spiritual care. As far as "pastoral care or psychotherapy?" is concerned, I appeal for a combination of these disciplines, also in one and the same person. Such a discipline might be called "therapeutically qualified pastoral care" or "psychotherapy that recognizes transcendence as the ultimate point of reference."

Psychotherapy

Over the past century, psychotherapeutic approaches and schools have greatly advanced the quality of caring, coping and "being with" (empathy), of methodological knowledge, and of awareness: Sigmund and Anna Freud, Carl Gustav Jung, Stanislav Grof, Fritz Perls, and Victor Frankl are just some of the pioneers. Creative and body therapies, as well as mindfulness, enhance self-perception and stress the importance of the individual moment, the *kairos*. Personally, I am committed to practicing psychotherapy with God/the Godhead as a final point of reference. This assertion is not based on scientific evidence, but on my personal experience with several hundred patients. It rests on a profoundly dialogic conception of the human person being related to others as well as to a greater and transcendent being. Given this characteristic of psychotherapy, I firmly believe in the transcendent, which we can experience as the primordial origin of our soul. This source nurtures, inspires, incomprehensibly carries, and serves as the existential basis of our primordial trust, just as it moves us toward a meaning and purpose of life. Such care is both psychotherapeutic and spiritual. Importantly, it involves a twofold concept of listening: first, listening to what our interlocutor's words say; second, listening to what lies concealed, unconsciously, behind utterances and asking ourselves and our intuition what is emerging into consciousness and searching for an answer. At the bedside of a critically ill patient, the spiritual caregiver attends to the here-and-now: a dream at night, a relationship problem, a restlessness almost unmanageable for the nursing staff. Some patients may need a family-therapeutic intervention, others music-assisted relaxation or a depth-psychological approach to a symbol or symptom. Spiritual caregivers, on the other hand, also inquire into an ongoing process: where is *this* patient in his or her inner maturation and dying process? Where does he or she get stuck? (see Renz 2015). *Indication-oriented* spiritual care goes beyond heeding verbally expressed patient needs. Understanding processes requires looking behind the symptoms, that is, understanding the conscious–unconscious dimensions along with patients' medical–clinical needs. Demand for efficiency is inevitable in everyday hospital life: illness, approaching death, the prospect of returning home, the family system, dreams, nightmares and anxieties all urge toward a process.

One classic example in this context is the loss of autonomy. It is important to share a patient's grief, as in the case of Sergio:

> *I empathized with him as far as possible, to understand what it must feel like if one can no longer walk, sit, speak or pass water. Anger and shame need enough space and freedom to find expression and also an utmost respect by all caregivers. Sergio, however, would not allow anyone near him, neither the nursing staff, nor his wife. The ward staff were exasperated. One day, I took the initiative and told this critically ill man emphatically about the dying process, about my experience with over a thousand dying patients, that their helplessness— if radically admitted—often turned into something beautiful, profoundly sensuous or spiritual, and that surely he did not intend to impede this process. "Aha," he uttered, as a sign of understanding. Could I tell him more? His wife recognized a pattern, a process. Already the next day, Sergio had managed to lose control of himself. Smiling, he stammered: "Flower, flowers." I felt reminded of the meadow in the folktale about Mother Hulda (see Chapter 4, footnote 3) and suspected a spiritual experience.*

Apart from our physical presence, therapeutic and spiritual care also needs interpretative and methodological skills to attend to the terminally ill and the dying (methods include imagination, dream interpretation, trauma therapy, music-assisted relaxation, body awareness exercises, focusing, dealing with transference and countertransference). Dream interpretation especially requires both a fundamental knowledge of symbols and metaphors and a well-developed sense of systematic methodology. Personally, I have found the work of Jung helpful, in particular his approach to dream interpretation and archetypal images; further, the approach of Grof; the knowledge of religion and shamanism gained as a student of theology and music ethnology; and finally my music therapeutic work with the body, sound and rhythm. In this approach to therapeutic-spiritual care spirituality sometimes remains dormant until, suddenly, it becomes important because of an unexpected experience of transcendence or because a patient wishes to pray. Experiences of transcendence need to be interpreted to become meaningful and develop their inherent energy. Sometimes, an *Aha!* moment happens and establishes that "more" has occurred than mere encounter or physical touch, more than a dream, more than music, relationship or a formal prayer—in other words, transcendence and grace. Even if, ultimately, everybody can reach a sound interpretation only by themselves, most patients need to be offered our intuitions. Our interpretations are a short- or long-term loan. Patients are allowed to accept or reject our loaned interpretation and gradually find their own. So much for my views and reflections on the therapeutic aspect of care.

Pastoral care

"Being there for the other." But is more than sheer presence involved? There are various models of hospital-based pastoral care. Speaking at a conference on pastoral care (Albisser 2010), Kunz distinguished three types of care: in the diaconic, solidarity-based approach, the pastor shares the patient's helplessness and speechlessness (Luther 1992); in the energetic-mystagogic approach, the pastor guides the patient toward a sacred place, for instance, through prayer, blessing and sacraments (Josuttis

2008); in the therapeutic-dialogic approach, the pastor listens to the patient's suffering and offers consolation (Klessmann 2009). These three approaches all involve empathic listening (Weiher 2012; Albisser 2010).

Both psychotherapy *and* pastoral care maintain the healing function of relationship. What, however, is the quality of a particular relationship, what is its atmosphere, and which capacity for encounter exists? Is the patient–caregiver relationship supported by specific techniques (e.g. imagination, music-assisted relaxation, prayer, meditation)? Atmospherically, this relationship needs to provide patients with the therapeutic freedom and space so that whatever needs to happen will happen. From this atmosphere there sometimes emerges that intense presence that is anything but passive: it contains the listening silence—the shared helplessness—and the space for the mystery of God and its ineffability. Explained in terms of Benedetti's approach to therapy (1992, 1998), this is "an existential togetherness." Benedetti accepts the need for boundaries, but also for their dissolution. He speaks of "partial identification," which occurs when therapists include aspects of a patient's suffering in their own experience while crossing the boundary (1998: 77–8). That is the core of empathetic suffering. On the patient–therapist relationship, Benedetti later added: "Opening up a part of ourselves to the patient while keeping the other part to ourselves is an essential problem" (Rachel 2000: 158). Ludwig Binswanger spoke of "carrying" (Bernhard-Hegglin 2000: 98).

Spiritual Care as Love and Alliance— Is that Asking too Much?

Love and existential togetherness take effect (see Chapter 6). Spiritual care in hospitals involves love capable of enduring and embracing suffering. By love, I mean a quality of compassionately being with, as well as accepting the other in his or her individuality. In such love, there is a time to perservere and a time to let go, to share joy and to share hopelessness. Love demands an autonomous personality capable of companionship and communion—with patients, with others, with God (Matthew 18.20). The capacity for love is a lifelong theme. To love, we must time and again reaffirm the other person, life, suffering and the ultimate, other dimension. Sölle (1993: 127–36) speaks of affirmation, that is, a fundamental attitude of positive assertion, but not of a fatalistic acceptance of suffering. For Rahner (1982: 175–6), affirmation is a basic decision: "There is total commitment, there is fundamental human decision, which remains anonymous and which one cannot grasp in material terms, nor judge or arrest, but that exists nevertheless." It could also be called loyalty, that is, an ultimate perseverance into apparent emptiness. Thus, one patient told me: "I can no longer love—but I can still be loyal, hour after hour." The same is true for many relatives and spiritual carers, whose contribution is modest and yet crucial. In lending our love to others, we share part of ourselves:

> *I accompanied Lawrence for two years. The hospital staff considered him a lost cause. I did not know why I made such an effort to engage in a therapeutic relationship with Lawrence. Perhaps because of a dream, in which I had carried this critically ill man in my arms, realizing that he could be "carried," that he was tolerable. Yet no ward was prepared to take him. His wife considered admitting him to a nursing home. In the beginning, our process intended to give him a chance—week after week, day after day. We formed an alliance: he promised to be constructive rather than cynical; his wife pledged that she would abandon the idea of a nursing home, at least for the time being; and the nursing staff and I promised that we would keep the faith and not give up on him. Despite this alliance, he repeatedly brought us to the brink of capitulation. Behind his aloof acerbity, I sensed despair. His situation was indeed desperate: never-ending illness, constantly diminishing mobility, a family unable to put up with him. I formulated my*

own despair with his cynicism and confronted him, but I kept my promise to stand by him. This moved him. After months in hospital, he was allowed home. His wife took him in once again. He tried to be constructive and experienced—as he put it—the "pinnacle of his life:" His family did not avoid him, he could look after the children, could walk almost upright and even ride a bicycle. Then his health declined again. He was readmitted to hospital and often sat in his wheelchair next to the hospital entrance feeding the birds. This was currently his joy of life, he told me. In between he grew bitter. Then he remembered his promise. Several days later, Lawrence lay on his deathbed and was no longer responsive. When I thanked him, I said: "Our alliance and arrangement stands: I believe in you, I trust you." He looked up at me, smiled, nodded, and then drifted away again. It was his last response. He died two days later.

It was never a matter of "love" between Lawrence, his wife, the hospital staff and myself. This was not a term we used. Essentially, his case amounted to perseverance instead of abandonment. Neither spirituality nor God was a subject of conversation. And yet I was not indifferent to his predicament. Here "alliance" occurred, from which grew a love of life, for his children, for birds, something stronger than his negativity. This alliance needs other human beings and even more—as my initial empowering dream had shown.

Like myself, the German theologian Dorothee Sölle (1993) advocated a more deeply-rooted love and affection, arguing that affirmation, as a fundamental human quality, runs counter to stoicism and indifference. The source of stoicism is "indifference, and no longer God; the absence of passion leads us to a supercillious coldness tinged with resignation" (27). Sölle, a fighter and rebel, acknowledged time and again the significance of vulnerability and a far from masochistic mysticism of the Cross: "The soul opens itself up to suffering. It gives itself to suffering and holds nothing back. It neither diminishes itself nor makes itself untouchable, nor does it distance itself or make itself insensitive. It allows itself to be completely affected by suffering" (128). "Christian religion affirms suffering in an almost incredible manner, more strongly than many other world-views not centered on the symbol of the Cross. This affirmation, however, is just one part of the great love of life" (135). According to Sölle, the path through the darkness of suffering leads us to a love that is actually an experience of God, of the ultimate. In her essay "Ich sehe das Leiden—ich glaube die Liebe" (I see the suffering—I believe in love), she wrote: "If the soul does not cease to love in the night of despair, 'into the void,' then the object of its love can justifiably be called 'God'" (1995: 218f.). Suffering makes us capable of loving, and lets our roots grow deeper and deeper. According to Richard Rohr, "pure presence" or "the naked now" and the freedom of "non-dualistic thinking" grow through serious suffering and through extreme loving (Rohr 2009: 122–8). Love brings into view human beings in their manifold suffering.

And yet can a person tormented by pain realistically still love—moreover into the void? Can the dying, can a relative, be asked to love a partner or a brother who leaves behind nothing but disappointment? Are the dying, by summoning all their willpower and physical strength, still capable of love, whereas in actual fact their tortured body seems deprived of a visible personality? What about us caregivers? Does the demand to love into nothingness—a love that endures and embraces suffering—not ask too much of us therapists, pastors, doctors, nurses, volunteers and relatives? Is existential togetherness not too great an imposition? What about our need for boundaries, what about self-love?

While we need to take these questions seriously, let me respond with another question: when is existential engagement in a relationship right, when is it mistaken? Perhaps listening to our inner voice is the only way of distinguishing compulsive self-sacrifice from an unconditional act of love. Neurosis rears its head all too quickly, urging us to escape from helplessness and to conceal our aggressions. Neurotic devotion, however, soon overwhelms us. Essentially, the unconditional act of love meant here amounts to being touched. Such love has time, and grants time. It also affords us the freedom to say "Yes" or "No." Ultimately, however, this love is genuine. Spiritual caregivers can decide only for themselves how intensely they choose to become involved with a patient. No sure formula exists, nor can one command "it" to be one way rather than another. We can only try to understand our motivation and limitations: what makes me engage so deeply with this person's fate, as if it were mine? To recognize this quality of love, we might ask: who do I love so much (my child, my sister, a particular woman or man) that I am inwardly driven to compassionate support for this person, of my own free will? This love is nothing that I can "produce." I can "want" it. It has to do with sympathy, beyond which it is something that happens: grace.

And yet, what helps spiritual caregivers cope with so much suffering, stress and distress? Speaking for myself, it is hope, regaining my will to hope time and again, and perseverance when, quite honestly, all that remains is loyalty. What helps me, too, are time-outs, nature, music, friendships and the study of the Bible. It is also important for my spiritual hygiene to accept that I am a human being with limited capacities. We hardly ever reach our goals, and that is allowed to happen. To step back is part of our authenticity. After my public lectures, I am often asked about experiences of failure, and my reply has to be: I fail everyday, here and there, and that too is permissible. What I find particularly helpful, however, are the workings of encounter: the risk of coming into contact, of touching and being touched inwardly. The only adequate and dignified way of reaching others is to make ourselves vulnerable and to risk being personally affected. From a radically dared encounter, we may emerge as a different person. In dealing with the critically ill, we must honestly ask ourselves: in such encounters it is not always clearcut who is the one who is doing the giving and who is receiving. Is it me who gives? Well, I offer music, my therapeutic skills, my time, sometimes even myself. Just as often, however, my patients give me something that, after our encounter, stays with me, enriches me and sometimes leaves a deep impression.

Patients enrich me with their presence, their testimony to bravery, their intense sensory impressions, their love, maturation and spirituality. It is precisely at the outermost limits of life that people find their way into a prayer that expresses something other than the faith they have been taught. Or they may discover a love distinct from common belief. Many patients are open to the suffering of others. They relativize their own pain by observing the fate suffered by others: patients who die young; children who are left behind; parents who lose a child. Being touched, patients ask me how *I* feel or, in their sleepless nights, they pray for others who are suffering. When asked about *themselves*, they are astonishingly capable of accepting their own fate. They are grateful for hours and simply "here," at times seemingly beyond time and space, and happy in that state, serene. Their many experiences of transcendence are unassuming and overwhelming at the same time. Taken seriously, patient testimonies suggest that an utmost experience of love involves something fundamental—called God, a supreme being or something else—that seems to exist no matter what. We are aware of such experience from the mystics, for instance, from Carmelite spirituality (for a discussion of bride mysticism, see Rotzetter 2000: 119–39). Spiritual care has to do with incomprehensible love and with mysticism.

Who Am I to Myself?—As a Prayer

Who am I? A person? An individual? Am I myself? A "you" to another? Am I searching for something, someone? Or am I, as Rahner would have it, a question asked "into endless obscurity"? In *The Need and the Blessing of Prayer*, in the chapter entitled "The Helper-Spirit," Rahner writes:

> Does today's man on his own really know more about himself than that he is a question into a limitless darkness, a question that only knows that the burden of questionability is more bitter than man can bear in the long run? (1997: 16f)

Do we find ourselves in the encounter with an ultimate, transcendent being? Defining our identity in relation to and determined by God or a supreme being, is uncommon nowadays. Our ego sees itself as the center of our self, our will, our actions, our feelings, in the midst of what we have become and our biography. I am who I am! The ego is the self-evident center of subject-related perception, which is so preeminent in the West. That is what is normal to our state of mind. However, human identity exceeds our ego. "Identity" raises perennial questions: who am I? And who am I meant to be? Identity develops or becomes obscured and assumes constantly changing guises. Identity is a relational term: we become through a Thou (Buber 1983), and, as I have hypothesized elsewhere, we die into an invisible Thou (Renz 2015). In the end, we are not an answer to ourselves. Bernhard-Hegglin (2000) speaks of "the dependence on being recognized by a Thou as an anthropologically constitutive element." Whether at the beginning of life or in its later stages, "being recognized… is the basis of our certainty of being…it is the source of every new beginning and of all development" (142–3).

Who or what, however, is that ultimate Other, which exists where there is no one but myself—in the midst of severe illness, utter abandonment, war, torture, existential poverty or private intellectual engagement? No one is spared this question and any answer already constitutes a decision: Bonhoeffer (1994) ends his famous poem "Who am I?" with the sentence: "Whoever I am, You know me, O God, I am yours!" (187). In his *Confessions*, the fourth-century Christian theologian Augustine

Hope and Grace

of Hippo (1914) wrote: "I beseech thee now, O my God, to reveal myself to me..." (X, 37). Paul the Apostle wrote the following words, which have lastingly—and controversially—influenced Western thought: "But by the grace of God I am what I am" (1 Corinthians 15.10). Today, and no differently than in the past, critically ill patients tell us that they feel deprived of their attractiveness, physical competence and other previously identity-establishing features. They are faced with the alternative of being nothing but a worm or finding their way ever more deeply into another identity. What emerges as a new sense of identity, as patients teach me time and again, is truer and more essential than what existed before. According to Rahner's approach to theology, their life can be seen as a new kind of prayer, in which patients are both: the question and the subject.

A German Jesuit priest and theologian, Karl Rahner (1904–84) devoted great attention to who we are. We face this question, which is at once real *and* inevitable, blankly, in the knowledge that we shall never escape from it nor find an adequate answer. It "brings us before ourselves," confronting us with the total sum of factors and lived experience (see Rahner 1984: 41–3). For Rahner (as already for Augustine[1]), this question—"Who am I?"—means that we are open to transcendence, standing firm on the one hand, surrendering on the other (1949: 18). Spending as much time as I do with the critically and terminally ill has helped me to understand Rahner's deeper concern. Over the years, I have ceased wondering about methods, but instead share patients' suffering and look for their deeper yearnings. This endeavor, in my eyes, forms part of a larger dialogue, as if I were to place the patient and his distress before God, the Godhead or the supreme being himself: "See...this is this particular person, his essential

---

1   Augustine of Hippo wrote in his autobiographical account *Confessions*: "I became a hard riddle to myself, and I asked my soul why she was so downcast and why this disquieted me so sorely" (IV, 4).

being, his suffering." Such a freely formulated prayer often has
the effect described by Rahner. Gathered in this prayer are a
patient's worries, emotions and tormenting questions. Therein
we are "brought before ourselves" and revealed onto ourselves
in our encounter with that unfathomable opposite. Thus, to
paraphrase Rahner, we are "the question I am to myself" (see
Rahner 1984: 41–3). Faced with this question, we stand firm
and also surrender. A prayer, which I always begin in a similar
way, has emerged from my professional practice:

> God/Godhead—whoever or whatever you are—here lies N.
> N., who is suffering very much. Come to us and be with us
> at day and at night, in the easy hours but especially in the
> difficult hours, even when we do not feel your presence.

Strangely, patients often breathe more freely during this prayer.
Also, they might add a word, cry, look at me or close their
eyes in worship. Here, then, something other than themselves
approaches them, to encounter not only their inner religious
child but also their present, incomprehensible self. They
might comment on this encounter as follows: "This is me.
HE has heard the prayer." "I have never experienced prayer
so truthfully." In prayer, patients become "more" than what
they have defined themselves as being so far. Even if we do
not pray "the question we are to ourselves" but merely live or
pronounce it, something essential happens nevertheless. For
instance, when patients feel ashamed and a burden to others,
and when we then express our esteem for them (in relation to
the absolute), they are astonished and feel dignified.

Even confused patients still have an identity and remain,
in their innermost, concerned with the meaning of their being.
I am often asked how I cope with patients suffering from
dementia. And I answer: what is truly essential occurs within
us. It is less important to visit such patients frequently than
to believe in their innermost, perhaps invisible, dignity and
identity. Such an attitude effects respect and reverence. Patients
suffering from dementia, patients with deliriums and patients

using terminal-stage symbolic language are relational beings and need an "opposite."

Gabriel, a dying man, took off all his clothes. For days, he lay on his bed naked. Although it was winter, he appeared to not feel the cold. Did he have another source of warmth? He wanted to return home, "to heaven," he told me. I was mostly looking after his wife, accompanying her on the difficult journey toward her husband's death. When, after several days, Gabriel still could not die, I interpreted his nakedness, in his wife's presence, based on account of Moses's experience of God at the burning bush (Exodus 3.1–12), as described by the German depth psychologist and exegete, Eugen Drewermann: "It is, of course, possible and necessary to enter paradise undressed, to come before one's maker unshamed and uninhibited. At a "sacred place," we are allowed to be as we are; we have nothing to hide...God...God is a God who wants and means the human being the way he is from his innermost nature" (1985: 386). Looking at Gabriel in his nakedness, I had to muster some courage to tell him about Moses. Then I said: "Perhaps you too are standing on holy ground and no longer need any covering. Whether naked or covered, you can be entirely yourself and come before God." To his wife's surprise and mine, Gabriel, who otherwise lay motionless on his bed, started stirring all over. He looked at us, groaned, and drifted away again, an astonished look on his face. "He understood that," his wife said, moved. Deep relaxation ensued, before Gabriel died peacefully an hour and a half later.

Chapter 9

Spiritual Care Interventions

Coping with Difficult Situations

Difficult situations abound in the context of illness. Difficulties arise partly from the specific nature of liminal experience (similar to the phenomenon of struggle discussed in Chapters 2 and 5). In everyday hospital life, fear—both specific and primordial—is an ever-present backdrop to patient symptoms, reactions and their specific fears (pain, darkness at night, abandonment, bodily symptoms like restlessness, sweating; see a list of concrete fears in Renz 1996/2009: 212–13). On the one hand, this book emphasizes understanding: understanding enriches and empowers us to provide competent and adequate spiritual care. For instance, understanding how profoundly sensitive patients are makes us mindful of their predicament and evokes our respect. Understanding how nurturing experiences of transcendence and other states of consciousness can be enhances our amazement and confidence.

On the other hand, this book highlights the need for continually raising and developing our awareness. Raising our awareness is different from understanding, it has to do with self-awareness and self-knowledge (e.g. of our hidden fears, motivations). Self-awareness enhances our caregiving skills. We always encounter patients as who we are. This is particularly important in regard to spirituality, as will be discussed in the next section. Here follows a list of spiritual care interventions:

- Listening and—as far as possible—being entirely with the patient while being ourselves. Being mindful of transferences and countertransferences as well as intuitions. At times, this may develop into existential togetherness.

- Normalizing: Under the particular circumstances, almost all patient reactions are normal and within the range of what might happen to us in their position. Anger, feeling overwhelmed and crying are normal. At times, a patient's inner world may be spinning, like a washing machine. I often explain the various stages of grief and loss to patients (and relatives).

- Listening between the lines: Certain information and certain situations need to be taken seriously while others may be consciously "overlooked." Should we feel overwhelmed, we may delegate responsibility to others, including God or the divine.

- Initiating subtle behavioral changes: Breathing consciously, bodily perception, relaxation; where necessary, summoning courage (with a dying patient, for instance, taking a leap of faith "into the unknown"). For instance, I often tell my patients to visualise how their body will be carried from the earth, and nobody fell through the earth from Europe to Australia.

- Being concise: Too many words overwhelm patients. Give our voices the significance they need. Listening to one's voice involves lifelong training: is our voice choked, subdued, impudent, or unrestrained (free), warm, present? The same applies to our appearance.

- Interrupting: Interrupting the other person's flow of desire, out of a need to retrace feelings, to breathe and to check for understanding.

- Centering: Repeating essential words and asking the patient to repeat them, combined in part with touch. (For instance, patients place their hand on their heart and feel themselves inwardly. Or we touch them.)

- Tell patients explicitly if we are going to touch them or move closer because, in the liminal sphere, every impression means "pressure" and may reactivate a traumatic experience. Any kind of contact and touch should be clearly communicated in advance.

- Ask "small" questions about the quality of life. For instance, "how are you sleeping?" "Did you see the tree in front of the window?" This experience of "my tree" during a critical illness in my youth is an experience of transcendence that I shall never forget.

- Is the patient having dreams? When interpreting dreams, remember that our interpretations and impulses are never final but "lent" to patients.

- Verbal expressions of confusion among the dying is often a lived language of symbols and as such more than "merely" delirious. Similar to dreams, this language is analogical and symbolically meaningful (for a list of metaphors, see Renz 2015).

- Use relaxation techniques, trauma therapy, active imagination.

- Make purposeful use of speech, singing and music.

- Intervention and confrontation based on experential knowledge: "Fear is not the ultimate truth"; "as much as I understand your resistance, ultimately you will find saying 'Yes' liberating." Often, I suggest that they try when they are on their own—when nobody is around and able to check—to say that difficult word "Yes." It is about having positive experiences.

- Spiritual differentiation between good and evil, between intentions and effects, between God/the good Godhead and demonic energies. Caregivers have to recognize negativity and destructiveness in patients, in the environment, and in themselves, even if they do not say anything. Recognition has two aspects: first, understanding how even these feelings have grown, and second rejecting them inwardly. Sometimes, expressing such distinction may also help. In this difficult issue, spiritual caregivers benefit greatly from spiritual exercises aimed at training such differentiations (e.g. contemplation) but also from psychotherapeutic processes: to recognize one's own shadow (Jung), to feel with the deprived inner child and integrate it, to be sensitive and even scared of one's increasingly uncontrollable negativity (negative energy, dream images of vortices and curses). This makes us modest and humble.

- As spiritual caregivers, we possess a great treasure of symbols, music, rituals (e.g. blessing), and perhaps even sacraments. But we have to implement these means carefully, knowing about the several layers of consciousness they may affect (see Appendix, Figures 10a and b). I have discussed the specific hearing sensitivity of terminally ill patients elsewhere (Renz 2015, Chapter 4).

- Consciously integrate the religious dimension when the situation suggests it. Every religious sign, gesture, prayer, sacred text and interpretation of an inner experience or a dream must be offered so that patients feel free to accept or reject it. In most cases, it is better to make a personal and genuine profession of faith rather than to shirk the issue (see below). In any case, it has to be pronounced in a way that patients feel free to agree or not. It is better to ask and not to avoid the omnipresent question of fate: why me? Why in this way? Expressing our indignation at a patient's fate is allowed.

• Be aware of the frequent reactivation of traumas in end-of-life patients. Sometimes, extra circumspection is called for, at other times committed love.

• Clear guidelines are often needed when dealing with relatives and difficult family circumstances. Importantly, we can normalize rather than pathologize a patient's condition, and we can give guidance to the relatives. who are often helpless. Even patients' and relatives' unusual behavioral patterns and coping strategies are normal in such situations. Distinguish patients and relatives according to their needs (who needs what?). Family taboos can be expressed cautiously.

• When we are dealing with patients who are dying, it is important to make their verbal, metaphorical, and nonverbal communication visible to relatives and to offer interpretations. Why the astonished look? Why the "death rattle"? Why the curled-up body? (see the list in Renz 2000/2008b). Our knowledge of near-death experiences helps relatives to understand that— inwardly—the dying are often elsewhere and that they are happy or serene in that state (Lommel 2010; Renz 2015). It is hardly a coincidence that precisely critically and terminally ill patients experience transcendence amid suffering. Understanding makes relatives feel pious and ceremonious.

• It comforts relatives to know that enduring suffering and the shock of seeing a loved one dying is an achievement. One young boy understood that coming to terms with his mother's imminent death was harder than climbing the Matterhorn, one of the highest mountains in the Alps.

How to Include God, Scripture and Religious Signs?

Spiritual care ought to be "spirituality-based." This self-evident statement is still not obvious: spiritual care is not identical with social care, with therapeutic, medical or nursing care. The spiritual focus entails the challenge of missing God/the Godhead/the divine, of looking for this hidden dimension, and of being sensitive to patients' experiences of transcendence. So how can spiritual caregivers make God/the Godhead and the sacred texts of any religion seem adequate and authentic so that this spiritual part of caregiving seems natural rather than not overly pious?

This question divides opinion. Those who secretly seek to convert others and who are therefore not free from an imposed compulsion, will also make the subtle impression of proselytizing. Those fixated on countering God and the churches, or those driven by the need to pander to trends and the *zeitgeist* also in spiritual matters will be perceived precisely in this way, thereby squandering their opportunity of discovering or admitting an autonomous, deeper-rooted spirituality. Religion and spirituality, moreover authentic spiritual care, can help patients connect with their own religious roots, verbally and non verbally. Credible spiritual care presents a challenge for *our* own maturation. Dare I take that freedom, just like Abraham, who—following the Lord's command—left his country? Dare I—time and again—forgive God, forgive the churches and their administrators? Only if I am free and committed solely to the absolute—called God, a supreme being, or an innermost authority—can I live and speak about my conviction and faith in a liberating, unimpeded way. This demands our personal, authentic spiritual path, our struggle with God, our experiences of grace, our knowledge of sacred texts, or relationship to them and scientifically grounded interpretations. Then, spiritual care opens up spaces where deep personal encounters and experiences of transcendence may happen—beyond the obvious needs of patients.

"What kind of God do you believe in?" Bernhard asked me between two bouts of pain. "I believe in the God that you need at this very moment," I replied spontaneously. He looked at me aghast and replied that if one felt as miserable as he did, it was best not to believe in any God at all. "I understand... that if there should be a God or a supreme being at all, then one who gives us freedom and also allows us not to believe." In his church, Bernhard continued, there had never been any mention of a God who lets people be as they were. He thought for a while: he had always imagined God as majestic, "but definitely not as a child in the manger, let alone a figure nailed to a cross." I remained silent. It was important to be allowed to have the freedom and the space to reflect. Answers would fall short and interrupt a process. We exchanged glances. For a moment, we remained silent and let time pass—were we allowed to spend this time? Then Bernhard wanted to know more. What exactly did I mean by was this "allowed"? I tried again: "If a God or a supreme being—then one who quite simply allows you to be." "But Mrs. Renz," he exclaimed, "if God exists, then surely he cannot leave me lying here in this misery!" But "precisely" this could also be God's distress, that he left human beings lying tormented on their deathbeds. This applied to him, here in Switzerland, just as much as it did to street children in São Paulo. Perhaps God wanted to tell us through Jesus, "I see eye to eye with you, I care about you." "But every religion has its own God and insists on being right." I took a deep breath. Bernhard felt my dismay, but he still wanted an answer. Could he remember the atmosphere of simply being allowed to be? "Oh, yes." "If there is a God, then he means this atmosphere. This is anything but self-righteousness. God

is much too great for us to have such a narrow view of him or to understand him at all." "Oh good." Finally, rounding off the if-God-statements, I said: "If God exists, then he exists also for you. I won't be talked out of believing that God is also here for you and that he can provide you with a profound answer." "Hm." That, for Bernhard, was the gateway to a deep personal experience of God (see Chapter 6).

Freda was pleased to be eating yoghurt again. Hospital life was dreadful, she said. No one had been to visit at Christmas, nor had she managed to reach out to a religious service from within herself. I was shaken. Was there a text or passage in the Bible that she particularly liked? "Oh, yes, simply Jesus." "As if separated from life," crossed my mind instinctively and the corresponding passage from the Gospel of Mark about the man with the withered hand (Mark 3.1–6). Jesus told the man to stand in the middle of those gathered. I shared this passage with Freda, adding that sometimes we felt as if our soul had to wither. "Yes, like here," she interrupted me. Could she manage to take her witheredness so seriously that she dared to stand in the middle, like the man in the synagogue? "What do you mean?" I guided Freda into relaxation and asked her to think of those hours when Christmas did not take place, of the emptiness and of the food that she did not like. Where did she feel withered within herself, where alive? Freda listened. "And now imagine Jesus were here, just as he was with that man in the synagogue." I prayed aloud: "Dear Jesus, this is Freda. She had a very hard time at Christmas." "Yes, everything was missing, there was no Christmas dinner, people were here, and yet they weren't." Then I played the harp. She began to cry, and I continued to play. Then I said: "Imagine Jesus had also told you not to be dead but to be alive, even if that is difficult in hospital." She cried even more intensely. I sang a well-known hymn ("Jesus, I Live to Thee"). The atmosphere became devotional. "Please sing the hymn again, HE is here," she asked me. Then there was silence. Would she like a Christmas

carol? She nodded. I sang "Silent Night." Deeply moved, she
said: "Christmas happened, just now."

How to Deal with Experiences of Transcendence

Do I believe in such experiences? This is the question that
experiences of transcendence by their very nature raise for
psychotherapy. The theological question is similar and yet
quite different: can experience be true and sacred even though
it corresponds neither to religious tradition nor to dogma?
Experiences of transcendence also remain a challenge after the
event, often urging us to engage with what has occurred and
find words for it, and to let such experiences resonate within
us, so that we actually recognize their sacred dimension. Does
our understanding of humanity and of God allow for such
experiences of transcendence? Can I permit such experiences to
touch me? How do we honor the holy in every experience and
religion within spiritual care without profaning the mystery
(see Neumann's discussion of Amor's warning to Psyche, 1981).
How do we identify the uniqueness of a patient's experience
without drawing premature conclusions from trends and from
our own conceptions? Is there room for such experiences in the
patient's terminology and our own?

Crediting an experience means recalling it time and
again. It is the purpose of religious rites and of the liturgy
to remember, observe and celebrate the mysteries on which
religions are founded. With my patients, I sometimes search
for memory objects (see also transitional objects; Winnicott
1953), for instance, a piece of music, an art postcard, or words
and phrases that sum up matters. Spiritual care, sometimes
even spiritual guidance, but also personal friendships, can be
vessels for the unfolding of spiritual experiences.

Regarding pastoral care and theology, it is worth
remembering that behind all religious tradition (and
dogma) there once stood an *experience* of God/the Godhead:

Revelation. For instance, from a human group's experience of liberation grew the people of Israel (from enslavement in Egypt to the crossing of the Red Sea, as depicted in Exodus). The overwhelming insight that "This is the work of God" (Exodus 15.21; condensed in Miriam's Song of Praise) formed the basis of religion and identity ("his people"). Before the rise of Christianity, Jesus, too, was a person and an "experience" shared by people at the time. Something similar occurs in individual experience: experiencing God establishes identity and "binds us back" (which is one of the two etymological meanings of "religion"; the other is reading again and remembering). The same happens to individuals today: they are deeply shaped by their experiences of the transcedent (see also Rotzetter 2000: 179). Does God reveal himself today, in the experiences of transcendence of individuals? Or do such experiences endanger the faith handed down for centuries? Experience, be it spiritual or not, is always personal. Sometimes, it coincides with (religious) traditions, at other times it does not.

The fear in the churches of religious and spiritual experience has been an important factor for centuries. It shows that the experience of God/the Godhead, the divine, has within it a subversive force. For instance, already Jeremiah was aware of the new autonomy of those who follow only the inner law (Jeremiah 31.31–4). This subversive aspect was also tangible in the force of liberation theology and the base ecclesial communities in the 1970s and 1980s. Part of this autonomy and force occurs in the existential being with patients, in touching, reflecting on their experiences of the holy and together feeling awe and wonder. Generally, spiritual experience gives rise to a strength that leaves behind distress, lethargy and fear! Spiritual experiences occur, either within or without a specific tradition, or beyond it. It leads to obedience and to utmost autonomy (see Introduction). Is this dangerous? Experiences of transcendence are not in themselves a matter of concern, although ill-considered (indifferent, fanatical and politically misguided) ways of dealing with such experience are.

The more we encounter grace, the more important our relationship with reality becomes. Can we protect and at the same time ground what we have been promised in our experiences of the holy? It is allowed and necessary for patients and caregivers to ask themselves time and again: What does this experience want to tell me? How can I transpose it into real life? What would I rather neglect, what would I deceive myself about? Safeguarding our relationship with reality may mean remaining silent about the core of the experienced mystery, as well as enduring the discrepancy between experience and reality, sometimes even to the point of leading a double life and, in its midst, having to wait for the *kairos* (the opportune moment; see Renz 1996/2009: 274–5: How can I go on living?). Part of such perseverance consists in finding our way back to everyday perceptions and values, and in accepting that life takes place primarily in the earthly, immanent dimension. Humility is part and parcel of every experience of transcendence, because it essentially exceeds everyday reality. Spiritual experiences do not strive toward escapism and addiction, but rather—through transformation and regeneration—toward a new responsible being in this world. In the image of the biblical story of the transfiguration of Jesus (Luke 9.28–36) we cannot abide at the site of extraordinary experience, nor build—as Peter suggested—tents around the ineffable. We must, instead, once again descend from the peak experience (from Mount Tabor), which also means drawing an even clearer boundary between God/the Godhead/the divine and humankind, between the sacred and the mundane. Fanatics, by contrast, act out their spiritual energy, tamper with the sacred and have an inflated perception of themselves (see Jung on the concept and temptation of inflation[1]). Grace remains a gift from God/the divine/a supreme being. It may approach us from outside or emerge from inside. It can arise from an ultimate ground and origin (Appendix, Figure 10a) or attract us from an all-embracing final end (Appendix, Figure 10b). We can, at best, experience and "understand" grace no more than in sudden breakthroughs and in fragments. As spiritual caregivers, we can pin our hopes on grace.

---

1 According to Jung, inflation involves the identification of the ego with the self, that is, the core of a human personality; inflation is rooted in dimensions that exceed the ego. Identification leads to megalomania and a sense of chosenness. Identification with the collective unconscious leads to archetypal contents invading the ego. In religious terms, this means that people want to be like God (see Hark 1988: 81f.).

Appendix

This Appendix presents the results of the research project "Spiritual experiences in suffering and illness," published in the *American Journal of Hospice and Palliative Medicine* as "Spiritual experiences of transcendence in patients with advanced cancer" (Renz *et al.* 2015).

Framework

All patients in my care were surveyed over a period of one year (see methodology and background research, as described in the Introduction). These patients were all suffering from late-stage cancer and undergoing shorter or longer treatment at our palliative-care or oncology unit. A total of 251 patients were observed. This amounted to approximately 25 per cent of all the patients hospitalized in both inpatient units (see Renz *et al.* 2015).

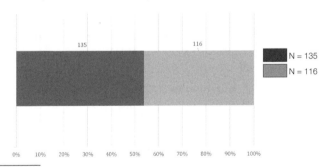

Figure 1: Frequency of spiritual experiences

Of the 251 patients, 135 described *one or more* spiritual experiences (see Chapter 4).

135 (53%) had one or several spiritual experiences

116 (47%) had no spiritual experiences or were unable or too shy to share their experiences

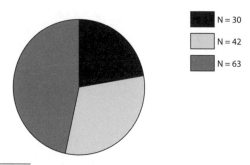

Figure 2: Experiences of transcendence and the time of death

Is there a connection between experiences of transcendence and being able to die? The patients studied were ill to varying extents. Life expectancy for many, even for patients receiving palliative care, was open. Some wanted to die, others did not. In both cases, death can occur faster and more suddenly than expected—or not. In our study:

N = 135 (100%)

30 patients (22%) of the patients surveyed were able to die within a few minutes or at the most within an hour (!) of (conveying) a spiritual experience; three patients died in the midst of such experience.

42 (31%) died within days or weeks of such an experience: either in hospital (30) or at home (12). In three (3) patients, the effects of spiritual experience (freedom from fear, absence of pain, altered sense of space, time and one's body) lasted for several days and remained until death.

63 (47%) returned to their everyday life (home, nursing home, home for the elderly) with a newly granted quality of life. They did not die within the survey year, but within two years after data collection began.

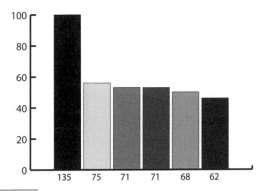

Figure 3: Associated reactions

Patients communicated numerous and significant effects of their spiritual experiences. Their quality of life and attitude toward life and death changed as follows:

N = 135 (100%)

135 (100%): altered sense of the present; a different, more intense bodily feeling

75 (56%): less fear; 15 patients had less difficulty breathing; 20 felt less nausea

71 (53%): pain relief

71 (53%): altered attitude toward life and (approaching) death

68 (50%): new attitude toward God/the divine, a new spiritual identity; these patients mentioned the term "God" at least once (9 of these patients were atheists/agnostics)

62 (46%): altered relationship to their illness

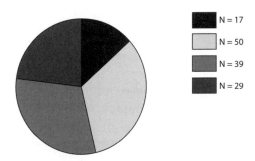

Figure 4: How long did the effects of such experiences last?

Figure 4 *cont.*

N = 135 (100%)

17 (13%): the experience faded again; 4 patients later denied having such an experience

50 (37%): a unique, unforgettable experience; initial experience

39 (29%): a recurring experience that grew deeper every time

29 (21%): the effects lasted several hours/days

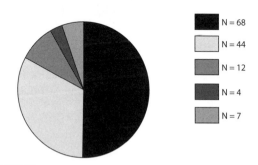

Figure 5: Religious affiliation

Spiritual experiences appear to influence religious identity (see Figure 3, indicating that 68 patients reported a new attitude to God/the divine). Is the opposite also true? No: our study demonstrates that spiritual experiences are not reserved for religious persons. The 135 patients in our study had different religious affiliations:

N = 135 (100%)

68 (49%): Catholic

44 (33%): Protestant, Evangelical

12 (9%): no religious denomination

4 (3%): Muslim

7 (5%): other

These religious affiliations corresponded to those of the population of Eastern Switzerland at the time of the survey.

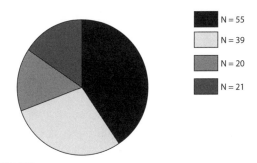

Figure 6: Religious attitude of patients

N = 135 (100%)

55 (41%): religion/church/religious community were important

39 (29%): estranged from their church, but seeking their own spiritual path and religious affiliation

20 (15%): agnostic/atheist

21 (16%): religious affiliation/attitude was not discussed

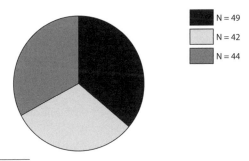

Figure 7: Previous spiritual experiences

Are previous spiritual experiences, for instance, in the context of near-death experiences, religious faith, meditation, spiritual crisis/psychosis, helpful? The 135 patients who had spiritual experiences included many *with* an earlier such experience, but also many without any at all.

Figure 7 *cont.*

N = 135 (100%)

49 (36%): first spiritual experience

42 (31%): previous spiritual experiences—

13 (10%) during meditation

25 (19%) during *experiences* of faith

11 (8%) previous near-death or similar experience

5 (4%) spiritual crises/psychosis

44 (33%): spiritual experiences were not discussed

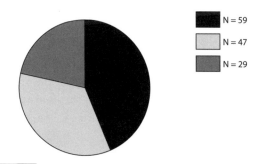

N = 59
N = 47
N = 29

Figure 8: How did patients communicate their spiritual experiences?

N = 135 (100%)

59 (44%): spontaneously reported all their spiritual experiences of their own accord.

47 (35%): reported at least *one* of their spiritual experiences while talking about themselves; in these cases, my questions helped patients to discover the moving, awe-inspiring, and spiritual nature of their experience.

29 (21%): could no longer form complete sentences because of illness and/or because they were deeply affected by the experience at least *once*. However, they unmistakably affirmed by stammering or nodding in recognition of the sacred nature of their experience and its possible effects.

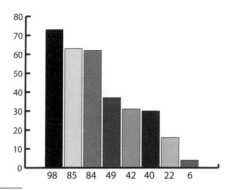

Figure 9: Preceding therapeutic and spiritual interventions/circumstances/inner experiences

N = 135 (100%)

98 (73%): music-assisted relaxation (Klangreisen)

85 (63%): religious support: prayers, blessing, sacraments, including—

49 (37%) wrestling with God

84 (62%): empathy, love

49 (37%): a solemn gathering of relatives at the bedside

42 (31%): dreams

40 (30%): maturation, reconciliation, integration of the dark sides of personality

22 (16%): presentiment of death/deathbed vision

6 (4%): remembering a previous near-death experience

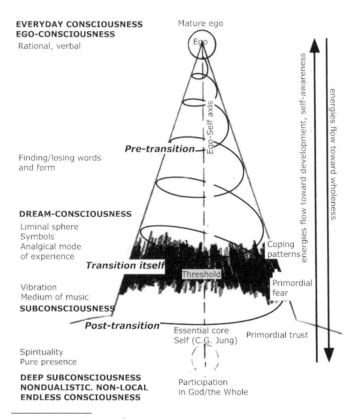

Figure 10a: States of consciousness

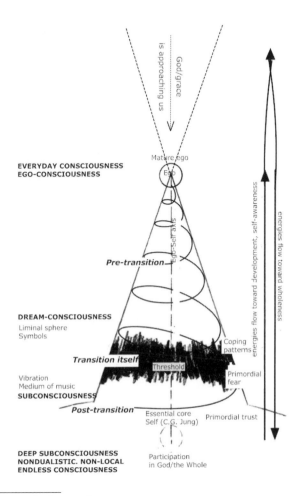

Figure 10b: States of consciousness

Table 1: Contents and types of spiritual experiences of transcendence

N = 135 (100%), multiple mentions possible

Periphery	Experiences in the liminal sphere of the sacred N = 116	Patients
	Angels, sacred atmosphere	66
	Forlornness, darkness, struggle	56
Center	Experiences of God/Being/Wholeness	
	"oneness" and Being/*unio mystica*	41
	an Other, "Otherness," a "Thou"	44
Center	Experiences of God/Being/Wholeness	
	God as father/mother	34
	"God/the divine in the midst" and amid suffering	33
	Spirit, energy	49
Total	Patients with spiritual experiences	135

References

Albisser, R. (2010) "Wofür stehe ich ein? Ökumenische Tagung der Spitalseelsorgenden." *Schweizerische Kirchenzeitung 178*, 13–14, 271–7.

Arnold, B. L. and Lloyd, L. S. (2013) "Harnessing complex emergent metaphors for effective communication in palliative care. A multimodal perceptual analysis of hospice patients' reports of transcendence experiences." *American Journal of Hospice and Palliative Medicine.* http://dx.doi.org/10.1177/1049909113490821

Augustinus (1914) *Des heiligen Kirchenvaters Aurelius Augustinus Bekenntnisse* (trans. Hofmann, A.) (Bibliothek der Kirchenväter, Bd. 1. Reihe 1, Bd. 18; Augustinus Bd. VII). www.unifr.ch/bkv/buch19.htm

Benedetti, G. (1992) *Psychotherapie als existentielle Herausforderung: Die Psychotherapie der Psychose als Interaktion zwischen bewussten und unbewussten psychischen Vorgängen und zwischen imaginativ bildhaftem und einschichtig begrifflichem Denken.* Göttingen: Vandenhoeck & Ruprecht.

Benedetti, G. (with Neubuhr, E., Peciccia, M. and Zindel, J. P.) (1998) *Botschaft der Träume.* Göttingen: Vandenhoeck & Ruprecht.

Bernhard-Hegglin, A. (2000) "Die therapeutische Begegnung: Verinnerlichung von Ich und Du." In B. Rachel (ed.) *Die Kunst des Hoffens: Begegnung mit Gaetano Benedetti.* Göttingen: Vandenhoeck & Ruprecht.

Bluebond-Langner, M., Belasco, J. B., Goldman, A. and Belasco, C. (2007) "Understanding parents' approaches to care and treatment of children with cancer when standard therapy has failed." *Journal of Clinical Oncology 25*, 17, 2414–19. http://dx.doi.org/10.1200/JCO.2006.08.7759

Bonhoeffer, D. (1994) *Widerstand und Ergebung. Briefe und Aufzeichnungen aus der Haft,* 15th revised edition. Gütersloh: Kaiser.

Breitbart, W., Rosenfeld, B., Gibson, C., Pessin, H. *et al.* (2010) "Meaning-centered group psychotherapy for patients with advanced cancer. A pilot randomized controlled trial." *Psycho-Oncology 19*, 1, 21–8. http://dx.doi.org/10.1002/pon.1556

Buber, M. (1983) *Ich und Du,* 11th revised edition. Heidelberg: Lambert.

Chochinov, H. M., Hack, T., Hassard, T., Kristjanson, L. J., McClement, S. and Harlos, M. (2005) "Dignity therapy. A novel psychotherapeutic intervention for patients near the end of life." *Journal of Clinical Oncology 23*, 24, 5520–5. http://dx.doi.org/10.1200/JCO.2005.08.391

Davies, S. L. (2002) *Gospel of Thomas: Annotated and Explained.* Woodstock, VT: SkyLight Paths.

Drewermann, E. (1985) *Tiefenpsychologie und Exegese. Bd 2. Wunder, Vision, Weissagung, Apokalypse, Geschichte, Gleichnis.* Olten: Walter.

Driedger, P. (2009) "Different lyrics but the same tune. Multifaith spiritual care in a Canadian context." In L. D. Bueckert and D. S. Schipani (eds) *Interfaith Spiritual Care. Understandings and Practices.* Kitchener: Pandora Press.

Fenwick, P. (2010) "Non local effects in the process of dying. Can quantum mechanics help?" *NeuroQuantology 8*, 2. www.neuroquantology.com/index.php/journal/article/view/281

Fenwick, P. and Brayne, S. (2011) "End-of-life experiences. Reaching out for compassion, communication, and connection-meaning of deathbed visions and coincidences." *American Journal of Hospice and Palliative Medicine 28*, 1, 7–15. http://dx.doi.org/10.1177/1049909110374301

Fenwick, P., Lovelace, H. and Brayne, S. (2010) "Comfort for the dying. Five year retrospective and one year prospective studies of end of life experiences." *Archives of Gerontology and Geriatrics 51*, 2, 173–9. http://dx.doi.org/10.1016/j.archger.2009.10.004

Frick, E. (2009a) "Seelsorge und Medizin. Spiritual Care: ein neues Fachgebiet der Medizin?" [Lecture 17 November 2009]. www.bayerische-stiftung-hospiz.de/pdf/Vortrag_DrFrick_Text.pdf

Frick, E. (2009b) "Spiritual care – nur ein neues Wort?" *Lebendige Seelsorge 60*, 4, 233–6.

Frick, E., Weber, S. and Borasio, G. D. (2002) "SPIR—Halbstrukturiertes klinisches Interview zur Erhebung einer 'spirituellen Anamnese'".

Fromm, E. (1976) *To Have or to Be: A New Blueprint for Mankind*. New York: Haper & Row.

Grimm (1984) *Kinder-und Hausmärchen gesammelt durch die Brüder Grimm. Bd. 1*. Frankfurt: Insel-Verlag.

Grof, S. (1991) *Geburt, Tod und Transzendenz. Neue Dimensionen in der Psychologie* (trans. Stifter, W.). Reinbek: Rowohlt. In English: (1985) Beyond the Brain: Birth, Death and Transcendence in Psychotherapy. Albany, NY: State University of New York Press.

Grün, A. (1993) *Biblische Bilder von Erlösung*. Münsterschwarzach: Vier-Türme-Verlag.

Grün, A. (2001) *Der Umgang mit dem Bösen. Der Dämonenkampf im alten Mönchtum,* 11th edition. Münsterschwarzach: Vier-Türme-Verlag.

Harding, S. R., Flannelly, K. J., Galek, K. and Tannenbaum, H. P. (2008) "Spiritual care, pastoral care, and chaplains. Trends in the health care literature." *Journal of Health Care Chaplaincy 14*, 2, 99–117. http://dx.doi.org/10.1080/08854720802129067

Hark, H. (1988) *Lexikon Jungscher Grundbegriffe. Mit Originaltexten von C. G. Jung*. Olten: Walter.

Herzka, H. S. and Jeanrenaud, M.-L. (1986) *Die Untersuchung von Kindern. Ganzheitliche Erfassung und psychischer Befund. Ein Leitfaden für den Untersucher*. Göttingen: Verlag für Medizinische Psychologie.

Herzka, H. S. and T. Reukauf, W. (1995) "Kinderpsychotherapie als dialogischer Prozess—ein der frühen Mutter-Kind-Entwicklung entsprechendes Konzept." In H. Petzold (ed.) *Die Kraft liebevoller Blicke: Psychotherapie & Babyforschung*. Paderborn: Junfermann.

Holder-Franz, M. (2012) *"Dass du bis zuletzt leben kannst. Spiritualität und Spiritual Care bei Cicely Saunders."* Zürich: Theologischer Verlag Zürich.

Holloway, M. A., Adamson, S., McSherry, W. and Swinton, J. (2011) "Spiritual care at the end of life. A systematic review of the literature." www.gov.uk/government/publications/spiritual-care-at-the-end-of-life-a-systematic-review-of-the-literature

Hommes, U. (1980) "Gespräch mit Manès Sperber." In U. Hommes (ed.) *Es liegt an uns. Gespräche auf der Suche nach Sinn*. Freiburg im Breisgau: Herder.

Hüther, G. (2001) *Biologie der Angst. Wie aus Stress Gefühle werden*, 6th edition. Göttingen: Vandenhoeck & Ruprecht.

Jäger, W. (2002) *Kontemplatives Beten. Einführung nach Johannes vom Kreuz*, 5th edition. Münsterschwarzach: Vier-Türme-Verlag.

James, W. (1979) *Die Vielfalt religiöser Erfahrung. Eine Studie über die menschliche Natur* (ed and trans. by E. Herms). Olten: Walter. In English: (1902) *Varieties of Religious Experience*. London: Longman Green.

Jaschke, J. (2013) "Gott fürs Gehirn—was die Neurobiologie über religiöse Erfahrungen sagt." *Christ in der Gegenwart 65*, 5, 61–2.

John of the Cross [Juan de la Cruz] (1987) *John of the Cross: Selected Writings* (ed. and trans. by K. Kavanaugh). New York: Paulist Press.

Josuttis, M. (2008) *Kraft durch Glauben. Biblische, therapeutische und esoterische Impulse für die Seelsorge*. Gütersloh: Gütersloher Verlagshaus.

Jung, C. G. (1961) *Erinnerungen, Träume und Gedanken* (ed. A. Jaffé). Zürich: Walter.

Jüngel, E. (1992) *Gott als Geheimnis der Welt. Zur Begründung der Theologie des Gekreuzigten im Streit zwischen Theismus und Atheismus*, 6th revised edition. Tübingen: Mohr. In English: (2014) *God as Mystery of the World*. London: Bloomsbury.

Kassel, M. (1980) *Biblische Urbilder tiefenpsychologischer Auslegung nach C. G. Jung*. München: Pfeiffer.

Keller, C. (2008) *On the Mystery Discerning Divinity in Process*. Minneapolis, MN: Fortress Press.

Keller, H. E. (2011a) "Mechthild von Magdeburg (1207–1282). Vom Fliessen des göttlichen Lichts." In A. Lutz (ed.) *Mystik. Die Sehnsucht nach dem Absoluten*. Zurich: Scheidegger & Spiess.

Keller, H. E. (2011b) "Meister Eckhart (um 1260–1328). Damit wir Gott Gott in uns sein lassen." In A. Lutz. (ed.) *Mystik. Die Sehnsucht nach dem Absoluten*. Zurich: Scheidegger & Spiess.

References

Kerr, C. W., Donnelly, J. P., Wright, S. T., Kuszczak, S. M., Banas, A., Grant, P. C. and Luczkiewicz, D. L. (2014) "End-of-life dreams and visions. A longitudinal study of hospice patients' experiences." *Journal of Palliative Medicine 17*, 3. http://dx.doi.org/10.1089/jpm.2013.0371

King, M., Llewellyn, H., Leurent, B., Owen, F., Leavey, G., Tookman, A. and Jones, L. (2013) "Spiritual beliefs near the end of life. A prospective cohort study of people with cancer receiving palliative care." *Psycho-Oncology 22*, 11, 2505–12. http://dx.doi.org/10.1002/pon.3313

Klessmann, M. (2009) *Seelsorge. Begleitung, Begegnung, Lebensdeutung im Horizont des christlichen Glaubens. Ein Lehrbuch.* Neukirchen-Vluyn: Neukirchener.

Klinger, E. (1994) *Das absolute Geheimnis im Alltag entdecken. Zur spirituellen Theologie Karl Rahners.* Würzburg: Echter.

Koenig, H. G., King, D. E. and Carson, V. B. (2012) *Handbook of Religion and Health*, 2nd edition. Oxford: Oxford University Press.

Kohut, H. (1979) *Die Heilung des Selbst.* Frankfurt: Suhrkamp.

Kraft, U. (2005) "Meditation. Die neuronale Erleuchtung." *Gehirn und Geist 10*, 12–17. www.gehirn-und-geist.de/alias/meditation/die-neuronale-erleuchtung/837043

Küng, H., Kuschel, K.-J. and Riklin, A. (2010) *Die Ringparabel und das Projekt Weltethos* (Kleine politische Schrifte, Bd 17). Göttingen: Wallstein.

Kunzler, M. (1998) *Amen, wir glauben. Eine Laiendogmatik nach dem Leitfaden des Apostolischen Glaubensbekenntnisses.* Paderborn: Bonifatius.

Lempp, R. and Becker, S. (1984) *Psychische Entwicklung und Schizophrenie. Die Schizophrenien als funktionelle Regressionen und Reaktionen.* Bern: Huber.

Lommel, P. v. (2010) *Consciousness Beyond Life. The Science of the Near-Death Experience.* New York: HarperOne.

Luban-Plozza, B. (2000) "Musik als Sprache der Seele." *Schweizerische Ärztezeitung 81*, 16, 838–40. www.saez.ch/docs/saez/archiv/de/2000/2000-16/2000-16-199.pdf

Luther, H. (1992) *Religion und Alltag. Bausteine zu einer praktischen Theologie des Subjekts.* Stuttgart: Radius-Verlag.

Lutz, A. (2011) *Mystik. Die Sehnsucht nach dem Absoluten.* [Museum Catalog, exhibition at the Museum Rietberg Zürich, September 23, 2011 to January 15, 2012]. Zurich: Scheidegger & Spiess.

Lutz, A., Greischar, L. L., Rawlings, N. B., Ricard, M. and Davidson, R. J. (2004) "Long-term meditators self-induce high-amplitude gamma synchrony during mental practice." *Proceedings of the National Academy of Sciences of the United States of America 101*, 46, 16369–73. www.pnas.org/content/101/46/16369.full.pdf%20html

McGrath, P. (2005) "Developing a language for nonreligious spirituality in relation to serious illness through research. Preliminary findings." *Health Communication 18*, 3, 217–35. http://dx.doi.org/10.1207/s15327027hc1803_2

Maslow, A. A. (1994 [1962]) *Psychologie des Seins. Ein Entwurf* (trans. Kruntorad, P.). Frankfurt am Main: Fischer-Taschenbuch-Verlag. In English: (1962) *Toward a Psychology of Being*. Princeton, NJ: D. Van Nostrand.

Mette, A. (2002) "Affinitäten postmoderner Religiosität zur hinduistisch-buddhistischen Spiritualität." *Religionen unterwegs. Zeitschrift der Kontaktstelle für Weltreligionen (KWR) in Österreich 7*, 3, 4–10.

Metz, J. B. (1975) "Unsere Hoffnung. Ein Bekenntnis zum Glaube in dieser Zeit." *Synode 2*, 84–111. www.weltanschauungsfragen.de/assets/Dokumente/Kirchliche-Verlautbarungen/03UnsereHoffnung.pdf

Neumann, E. (1960) "Das Schöpferische als Zentralproblem der Psychotherapie." *Acta Psychotherapeutica et Psychosomatica 8*, 351–64.

Neumann, E. (1981) *Amor und Psyche. Deutung eines Märchens. Ein Beitrag zur seelischen Entwicklung des Weiblichen*, 3rd edition. Olten: Walter.

Nouwen, H. J. M. (2007) *Du bist der geliebte Mensch. Religiös leben in einer säkularen Welt.* Freiburg im Breisgau: Herder. In English: (1992) *Life of the Beloved: Spiritual Living in a Secular World* (trans. Schellenberger, B.). New York: Crossroad.

Otto, R. (1987 [1917]) *Das Heilige: Über das Irrationale in der Idee des Göttlichen und sein Verhältnis zum Rationalen. (Nachdruck der Ausgabe 1979).* Munich: Beck. In English: (1958) *The Idea of the Holy*, 2nd edition. New York: Oxford University Press.

[183]

Puchalski, C., Ferrell, B., Virani, R., Otis-Green, S., Baird, P., Bull, J. and Sulmasy, D. (2009) "Improving the quality of spiritual care as a dimension of palliative care: the report of the Consensus Conference." *Journal of Palliative Medicine 12*, 10, 885–904. http://dx.doi. org/10.1089/jpm.2009.0142

Rachel, B. (2000) *Die Kunst des Hoffens. Begegnung mit Gaetano Benedetti*. Göttingen: Vandenhoeck & Ruprecht.

Rahner, K. (1949) *Von der Not und dem Segen des Gebetes*. Innsbruck: Rauch. In English: (1997) *The Need and the Blessing of Prayer* (trans. Gillette, B.). Collegeville, MN: Liturgical Press.

Rahner, K. (1960) "Zur Theologie der Menschwerdung." In K. Rahner (ed.) *Schriften zur Theologie: Bd. 4*. Einsiedeln: Benziger.

Rahner, K. (1969) "Meditation über das Wort Gott." In H. J. Schultz (ed.) *Was ist das eigentlich—Gott?* (Die Bücher der Neunzehn: Bd. 119). Munich: Kösel.

Rahner, K. (1982) *Praxis des Glaubens. Geistliches Lesebuch* (eds A. K. Lehmann and A. Raffelt). Freiburg im Breisgau: Herder.

Rahner, K. (1984) *Grundkurs des Glaubens* (Sonderausgabe). Freiburg im Breisgau: Herder.

Rahner, K. (2004) *Von der Unbegreiflichkeit Gottes. Erfahrungen eines katholischen Theologen*. Freiburg im Breisgau: Herder.

Reiterer, F. V. (2009) "Gott." In F. Kogler and R. Egger-Wenzel (eds) *Herders neues Bibellexikon*. Freiburg im Breisgau: Herder.

Renz, M. (2007) *Von der Chance, wesentlich zu werden. Reflexionen zu Spiritualität, Reifung und Sterben*. Paderborn: Junfermann.

Renz, M. (2008a) *Erlösung aus Prägung. Botschaft und Leben Jesu als Überwindung der menschlichen Angst-, Begehrens- und Machtstruktur* (Dissertation, Universität Fribourg). Paderborn: Junfermann.

Renz, M. (2008b [2000]) *Zeugnisse Sterbender. Todesnähe als Wandlung und letzte Reifung*, 4th revised edition. Paderborn: Junfermann.

Renz, M. (2009 [1996]) *Zwischen Urangst und Urvertrauen. Aller Anfang ist Übergang. Musik, Symbol und Spiritualität in der therapeutischen Arbeit*, 2nd revised and extended edition. Paderborn: Junfermann.

Renz, M. (2010 [2003]) *Grenzerfahrung Gott. Spirituelle Erfahrungen in Leid und Krankheit*. Freiburg: Kreuz.

Renz, M. (2013a) *Der Mystiker aus Nazaret. Jesus neu begegnen. Jesuanische Spiritualität*. Freiburg: Kreuz.

Renz, M. (2013b) Religionen sind eine existenzielle Antwort—doch worauf? *Neue Zürcher Zeitung, 23*.

Renz, M. (2014a [2011]) *Hinübergehen. Was beim Sterben geschieht. Annäherungen an letzte Wahrheiten unseres Lebens*. Freiburg: Kreuz.

Renz, M. (2014b) *Hoffnung und Gnade Erfahrung von Transzendenz in Leid und Krankheit—Spiritual Care*. Freiburg im Breisgau: Kreuz.

Renz, M. (2015) *Dying: A Transition* (trans. Kyburz, M. with Peck, J.). New York: Columbia University Press.

Renz, M., Schuett Mao, M., Bueche, D., Cerny, T. and Strasser, F. (2013) "Dying is a transition." *American Journal of Hospice and Palliative Medicine 30*, 3, 283–90. http://dx.doi. org/10.1177/1049909112451868

Renz, M., Schuett Mao, M., Omlin, A., Büche, D., Cerny, T. and Strasser, F. (2015) "Spiritual experiences of transcendence of patients with advanced cancer." *American Journal of Hospice and Palliative Medicine 32*, 2, 178–88. http://dx.doi.org/10.1177/1049909113512201

Riedel, I. (1989) *Die weise Frau in uralt-neuen Erfahrungen. Der Archetyp der alten Weisen im Märchen und seinem religionsgeschichtlichen Hintergrund*. Olten: Walter.

Rohr, R. (2009) *The Naked Now. Learning to See as the Mystics See*. New York: Crossroad.

Roser, T. and Borasio, G. D. (2008) "Der Tod als Rahmenbedingung. Spiritual care in der Palliativmedizin." *Praktische Theologie 43*, 43–51.

Rotzetter, A. (2000) *Spirituelle Lebenskultur für das dritte Jahrtausend*. Freiburg im Breisgau: Herder.

Rusterholz, S. (2011) "Jakob Böhme (1575–1624). Als Ketzer verdammt verehrt als Mystiker und philosophus teutonicus." In A. Lutz (ed.) *Mystik. Die Sehnsucht nach dem Absoluten*. Zurich: Scheidegger & Spiess.

References

Rutishauser, C. M. (2013) "Interreligiöse Kompetenz nötig. Gerade die heutige Welt braucht den Dialog der Deutungssysteme." *Neue Zürcher Zeitung,* 16. www.nzz.ch/meinung/debatte/vielfalt-fruchtbar-machen-1.18210321

Ruysbeek, E. v. and Messing, M. (1999[1990]) *Het Evangelie van Thomas.* Utrecht: Uitgeverij AnkhHermes.

Scagnetti-Feurer, T. (2009) *Himmel und Erde verbinden. Integration spiritueller Erfahrungen* (Dissertation, University of Zurich). Würzburg: Königshausen & Neumann.

Schnabel, U. (2002) "Die Biologie des Glaubens. Mystische Erlebnisse auf Knopfdruck." *Geowissen* 3, 31–40.

Schwager, R. (1996) *Jesus im Heilsdrama. Entwurf einer biblischen Erlösungslehre,* 2nd edition. Innsbruck: Tyrolia.

Sölle, D. (1993) *Leiden.* Freiburg im Breisgau: Herder. In English: (1975) *Suffering.* Philadelphia, PA: Fortress.

Sölle, D. (1995) "Ich sehe das Leiden—ich glaube die Liebe" In R. Walter (ed.) *Leben ist mehr.* Freiburg im Breisgau: Herder.

Steinhauser, K. E. and Barroso, J. (2009) "Using qualitative methods to explore key questions in palliative care." *Journal of Palliative Medicine 12,* 8, 725–30. http://dx.doi.org/10.1089/jpm.2009.9580

Sudbrack, J. (1999) *Gottes Geist ist konkret. Spiritualität im christlichen Kontext.* Würzburg: Echter.

Sulmasy, D. P. (2002) "A biopsychosocial-spiritual model for the care of patients at the end of life." *The Gerontologist 42* (Spec No. 3), 24–33.

Sulmasy, D. P. (2006) *The Rebirth of the Clinic. An Introduction to Spirituality in Health Care.* Washington, DC: Georgetown University Press.

Teilhard de Chardin, P. (1959 [1955]) *Der Mensch im Kosmos* (trans. Marbach, O.). Berlin: Union-Verlag. In English: (1959) The Phenomenon of Man. New York, NY: Harper & Brothers.

Weiher, E. (2012) "Spirituelle Begleitung in der Palliativmedizin." In E . Aulbert, F. Nauck and L. Radbruch (eds), *Lehrbuch der Palliativmedizin,* 3rd edition. Stuttgart: Schattauer, 1149–71.

Wilber, K. and Wilber, T. (1996) *Mut und Gnade. In einer Krankheit zum Tode bewährt sich eine grosse Liebe* (trans. Eggert, J.) 16th edition. Munich: Goldmann. In English: (1992) Grace and Grit: Spirituality and Healing in the Life and Death of Treya Killam Wilber. Boulder, CO: Shambhala Publications.

Winnicott, D. W. (1953) "Transitional objects and transitional phenomena. A study of the first not-me possession." *International Journal of Psychoanalysis 34,* 2, 89–97.

Winter, H. (May 10, 2013) "Unterschiede hervorheben statt einebnen." *Neue Zürcher Zeitung,* S. 21. Abgerufen. www.nzz.ch/meinung/debatte/unterschiede-hervorheben-statt-einebnen-1.18078633

Zaehner, R. C. (1980) *Mystik: Harmonie und Dissonanz: die östlichen und westlichen Religionen* (trans. Benz U. and Braun, H.-J.). Olten: Walter.

Subject Index

Author Index